Praise for *Pets and the City*

"Dr. Amy visits her patients in their New York City habitats: the grand (and sometimes not-so-grand) homes and apartments where they live. These stories feel like you have hopped into her leather doctor's bag and gone along for the ride, getting a peek at the houses and lifestyles of the people while learning about the pets she doctors. This book is a treat for anyone who ever wanted to be a vet—and those who are curious how the rich (and their pets) are different from us."

—Tracie Hotchner, author of *The Dog Bible* and *The Cat Bible*

"A lovely, compelling memoir written with humor, honesty, and personal drama . . . This is an engaging and well-told true story."

—Lee Gutkind, author of *The Fine Art of Literary Fist-Fighting*

"Dr. Attas is part doctor, part educator, part counselor, and all heart—caring not just for pets but for their people. This waggish memoir follows her from mansions and penthouses to studio walk-ups as she performs one of the toughest and most rewarding jobs: protecting our best friends, in every season of life."

—Laurie Zaleski, author of
Funny Farm: My Unexpected Life with 600 Rescue Animals

"Dr. Attas's warm and wonderful *Pets and the City* is New York City's version of *All Creatures Great and Small*. Whether she's treating the ailing cat of a hoarder in a tiny apartment or a super model's diseased Pekingese on Park Avenue, her compassion, humor—and affection—for people and their pets shines through. The perfect beach read for animal lovers."

—Cat Warren, *New York Times* bestselling author of
What the Dog Knows

Pets

and the

City

True Tales of a Manhattan
House Call Veterinarian

Dr. Amy Attas

Founder of City Pets

G. P. Putnam's Sons
New York

PUTNAM
—EST. 1838—

G. P. PUTNAM'S SONS
Publishers Since 1838
An imprint of Penguin Random House LLC
penguinrandomhouse.com

Hardcover ISBN: 9780593715673
Ebook ISBN: 9780593715680

Printed in the United States of America
1st Printing

All of the stories in *Pets and the City* were inspired by my memories of actual events. In some cases, I have taken the liberty of changing names, addresses, and identifying characteristics of some pets and their owners.

For my husband, Steve,
my partner in everything

Contents

Introduction

Conversation stops at Manhattan dinner parties when someone asks me, "So what do *you* do?"

"I'm a veterinarian."

At least one person then exclaims, "That's what *I* always wanted to be!"

Same, I think. I was the kid who gave injections to my stuffed animals and wrapped ACE bandages around my pet dog's neck until my parents made me stop.

Now I *am* a veterinarian, and it's everything I'd ever hoped it would be. Better, in fact, because in my case, I don't work with dogs and cats in a sterile hospital or clinical environment. Instead, I make house calls and treat the pets where they live—in penthouses, apartments, and walk-ups—all over Manhattan.

I not only get to treat the animals I love . . . I also get to peek into their owners' lives, as well. For a lifelong New Yorker like me, the privilege of doing this job in this city is like hitting the jackpot.

I've been on this path since September 1992, when I came up

with the idea for City Pets, Manhattan's first full-time veterinary house call practice. Nothing like it existed back then, so I developed the business plan as I went along. Right from the start, I booked four, six, and sometimes eight appointments per day. On any given workday, my assistant and I would travel from Battery Park City at the bottom tip of Manhattan to Harlem up top, from the East Side to the West Side, going into the homes of the superrich—and those just getting by. Throughout it all, I've had a front-row seat to the private and secret lives of New Yorkers and their pets.

Then and now, each day starts with a schedule of appointments, listing the names and addresses of the pets, their families, and what each animal needs that day. After loading the necessary equipment and medications into wheelie suitcases, tote bags, and backpacks, my nurse and I set off with a tentative plan . . . one that is constantly changing due to last-minute emergencies or calls about sick pets who can't wait. It's hectic, frenetic, and nerve-racking work. It's also incredibly exciting.

A typical day at City Pets looks something like this.

My first patient of the morning was Biscuit Roseton, a white Jack Russell terrier with fawn spots and floppy ears who, despite her problems, always had a friendly smile on her face. She lived in a huge, five-story Beaux Arts mansion on the Upper East Side, which was a treat to visit in its own right.

I'd been visiting Biscuit five days each week for over six months because she needed special attention. Her owner, Mrs. Roseton, had backed her car out of the garage of the family's Southampton mansion and accidentally ran over Biscuit's hindquarters. Although Biscuit had been whisked to an emergency hospital for life-saving care, her spinal cord had been severely damaged and the family was told that she would never walk again. That's when Mrs. Roseton called me.

My physical therapy with Biscuit had been going well—she would never regain full mobility, but my goal was to build up her strength sufficiently to allow her to use a two-wheel cart to get around. To accomplish this, my assistant George and I would fill the huge Jacuzzi tub in the Rosetons' master bathroom with warm water and place Biscuit in it, her front legs draped over the tub's reading tray like a kickboard and her back legs dangling in the water. With the tub's sixteen jets creating a stimulating whirl, I'd manipulate Biscuit's rear legs underwater around and around like she was riding a bicycle. George kept Biscuit's attention by feeding her delicious, tiny pieces of treats.

And it was working! Biscuit loved these half-hour Jacuzzi physical therapy sessions (or maybe just the treats), and after a week or so her muscle tone had visibly improved. After three months, she could partially stand with assistance. At five months, I saw evidence of spinal walking, an involuntary movement that mimics a natural step even though there is no communication between the brain and the legs, like a drunken drag. It's not pretty, but it is independent motion.

I was excited to track any new improvement at today's visit. I rang the doorbell and was let in by a discombobulated Mrs. Roseton. "Dr. Amy! I'm sorry, I should have called and canceled today's visit," she said.

The usually impeccable townhouse was in complete disarray. Water rained down the spectacular central grand staircase like a circular Niagara Falls. Half a dozen people were rushing around the lobby vacuuming up the water and trying to get the flooding under control.

"What happened?" I asked.

"The pipes burst! The plumber said the drain in the master bathroom Jacuzzi was hopelessly clogged, and when the pipe burst, water poured all the way down to the basement."

George and I looked at each other and gulped. Jack Russell dogs shed prodigiously and no one—including me—had thought to clean the fur out of the drain after each of Biscuit's physical therapy sessions. Five months of daily PT had produced a lot of fur.

I couldn't help thinking, *This is my fault; I hope she isn't going to fire me.* I wanted to follow through with Biscuit and, to be honest, I needed Mrs. Roseton's business.

"*There* she is!" said Mrs. Roseton. Her stressed expression went back to her usual smile when she saw little Biscuit stumble-walk over to greet us in the chaotic lobby with her Jack Russell smile on her face. It was clear that Mrs. Roseton didn't care about the tens (hundreds?) of thousands of dollars of water damage I had caused—only that Biscuit was now able to get around.

She beamed at Biscuit and turned to me, "We shouldn't waste a session. Can you work in the kitchen today? It's the only dry room in the house."

"We'll figure something out," I said, trying to not show how relieved I was that she didn't boot me out the front door.

Our next appointment was on East 26th Street and Lexington Avenue in the Flatiron neighborhood—and it couldn't be more different from the grandeur of Biscuit's marble-clad townhouse. Gail was a new client, and she'd scheduled a visit for Sweetie, her ten-year-old gray-and-white cat who was suffering from constipation.

It took a full half hour to get the few miles downtown, and we arrived at a nondescript apartment building with about fifty units. I rang the exterior buzzer, and we were let through the two front doors. We walked down a dark, narrow corridor to the elevator, which was making grinding noises as it descended toward the lobby.

"I'm not getting in that thing," declared George. "It's a death trap!"

I rode up to the fifth floor with our equipment, and he ran up the five flights of stairs. He was huffing and puffing as we walked through a dimly lit warren of hallways, until we found 5F and rang.

A heavy-set, braless middle-aged woman in an oversized *Simpsons* T-shirt and torn leggings was trying to open her apartment door wide enough so we could come in. "I guess that's as far as it goes," Gail said, unfazed. I squeezed through the opening but had to turn my wheelie suitcase sideways to get it through.

Once inside, I saw why Gail couldn't open the door all the way. There were stacks and stacks of newspapers and other detritus on the floor behind the door.

Gail was a hoarder. Her one-bedroom apartment was crammed with a lifetime of things that should have been thrown out years before. We followed her along a narrow passage between piles of papers, torn cardboard boxes, and stacks of milk crates she'd pulled in from the street to hold things.

Everywhere I looked were dirty clothes, jars with mysterious contents, and piles of unwashed dishes. It smelled like decay with a hint of marijuana. On the floor of the kitchen, I saw dozens of small bowls with remnants of crusty canned cat food that had been offered to Sweetie days or even weeks before.

Sweetie circled Gail's legs. She was a handsome white cat with gray spots who was in serious need of grooming. "I think she's constipated," said Gail, as she pushed her frizzy silver hair behind her ears.

"Let's see what's going on," I said. Ready to do the exam, I looked around the cluttered living room for a clear space to set up, but every flat surface was covered with some kind of debris. Gail was sitting on the only free chair.

"Do you have a table I can work on?" I asked Gail.

She looked around and concluded, "No."

"Where do you eat?"

"I eat standing up."

Okay. George and I moved some boxes and made a space to work on the dusty floor, which I was reluctant to kneel on. Sweetie's physical exam was normal, and she was not constipated. In this chaotic mess of an apartment, she could have defecated anywhere, and it would have been impossible to find. I took some blood tests, got her up-to-date on her vaccines, trimmed her nails, and combed through her fur, apparently for the first time.

"Can you show me her litter box?" I asked.

"In the bathroom, over there." Gail pointed the way.

George stayed with Gail while I ventured forth. The bathroom was truly squalid. Stains on the floor, on the walls, inside the toilet; clumps of hair in the drains (paging Mrs. Roseton's plumber); and truly the most disgusting litter box I'd ever seen. It was filled almost to the top with hundreds of little hard stools, and from the look and smell of it, Gail hadn't cleaned the box in months.

How could she possibly tell whether her cat was constipated when she didn't scoop the litter box?

I returned to the living room to find Sweetie sitting on Gail's lap and rubbing her face against her owner's cheek. Gail gave her companion a kiss and smiled for the first time at us. "Thanks, Doc, she looks better already."

These two were clearly in love with each other.

"Gail, there are a few things that I need you to do to keep

Sweetie healthy. Give her fresh cat food and water *every day*. Pick up the bowls afterward *and wash them*. Very, very important: clean her litter pan *daily* so you know exactly when she is defecating."

"I will, Doc."

"I'd like to see her again in a month." Maybe if Gail knew I was coming back, she'd be vigilant about the fresh cat food and litter maintenance.

Gail agreed, and I felt relieved. This way, I would be able to keep an eye on them both, as it seemed the patient *and* the client needed a bit of help. At that moment, I didn't know how prescient my thoughts were.

We were running late for our next appointment in Chelsea, at the home of a husband and wife who were international stars in the classical music world. With most of my married-couple clients, I dealt with the wife. However, things were reversed at the Hurvitz household.

"Schumann has a sick stomach," said Mr. Hurvitz as soon as he opened the door, handing me the leash of his spaniel before I'd even crossed the threshold.

"He's *fine*," Mrs. Hurvitz corrected from the other room. "He just ate too much and puked."

"When did this happen?" I asked.

"Yesterday morning," said Mr. Hurvitz.

"Has he vomited since then?"

"No, and he ate all his meals and then some, with no more vomiting. I even gave him my bagel this morning."

"Any diarrhea or soft stool?" I continued.

"No. All of that is normal."

"Have there been any other symptoms?"

"No, but you can never be too careful," he said.

Mrs. Hurvitz had come into the room and was annoyed. "Mindel," she said to her husband, "in eighteen years you never went to a single pediatrician appointment for our son. Not for a routine checkup and not even when he was sick, and now you have the vet on speed dial!?"

"I love my dog!" he rebutted.

The house calls I made that morning were to just a handful of the more than 7,000 Manhattan families and their 14,000 pets that I've made since I started my house call practice. Some were one-time-only visits, but most of my client families have been with me for years or even decades. I meet many of them right when their new pet babies come home, and see them through puppy- and kittenhood, giving them their vaccinations, treating their ear infections and stomachaches, and providing years of general wellness care. I treat their ailments as they become adults and seniors. And, sadly, when it is time, I put those same cherished pets to sleep.

I see the full cycle of life of both my patients and their families.

Because of what I've been exposed to, I've learned a lot about human nature. For example, what people show to the world is not necessarily who they really are. I've had clients who dressed like messy high school students in ripped jeans and ratty T-shirts and was then stunned to find out they lived in a $9 million duplex on Fifth Avenue (with a second home in Aspen). I've also seen the reverse: an all-designer-all-the-time publicist to the stars who lived in a tiny, rent-controlled studio in Alphabet City. She spent all her money on her clothes—and her cats.

I am also privy to the intimacies and true nature of my clients' lives. The things people leave out even when they know we're coming—porn, intimate letters, bank statements, stacks of cash, jewelry, adult toys—never ceases to amaze me.

If I worked in a brick-and-mortar animal hospital, I wouldn't see any of that. I wouldn't learn what's really going on in the pets'—or their owners'—lives, or about their bonds with their pets. And I wouldn't develop the close relationships with my clients that I have.

When I first met Mrs. Roseton, for example, she was utterly distraught about accidentally injuring her dog. But by showing up every day to help restore muscle strength in Biscuit's legs, I was also giving Mrs. Roseton hope and a sense of agency. She never even mentioned that we were the culprits who flooded her gorgeous home—instead, we were the heroes who returned to her a dog with a good quality of life and so assuaged her guilt over the accident.

When I saw Gail's atrocious living conditions and returned again and again, I knew that our work was not only to check if Sweetie was constipated but also to ensure that Gail remained healthy in body and mind. Because Gail trusted me to enter her unique space and by continuing to show up regularly at her apartment, I kept track of her physical and mental health, too. In fact, for quite some time, I am pretty sure I was the only health care professional she had any contact with. In a way, I worked alongside Sweetie to keep Gail functioning. And when Sweetie herself got sick, my team and I stepped up in a big way for both of them, because we knew how high the stakes were.

To the outside world, the Hurvitzes were the perfect cultural power couple. But I saw something else. I believe Mr. Hurvitz was free to express his love for Schumann in a way that he was never able to with the rest of his family, and I think they were jealous of that. How we treat our pets often reveals strengths and weaknesses in our other relationships.

I was born a New Yorker and born to be a veterinarian. I've devoted my life to serving the dogs and cats in the city that I love. I've fulfilled my James Herriot *All Creatures Great and Small* dreams of traveling to people and pets where they live and becoming an integral part of their lives. Early on, I thought that my calling was simply to learn about and care for animals in a sterile hospital setting, but I now know that is a narrow view of what my profession should be.

I care for the animals that belong to people—and, by extension, I care for the people as well. I love both aspects of my work.

And whether I'm trimming a billionaire's cat's nails or chatting with the building's doorman about his dog's limp, I treat every client the same, because each one of them loves their pets wholeheartedly. Love knows neither rank nor bank account. I've been a witness to the love between all types of people and their pets every day of my working life for over thirty years, and it has been a privilege.

On these pages, I'm sharing some of my experiences that reveal basic human truths about the power of the special bond between people and their pets, about the importance of animals in our lives, and about the complexities of human nature.

A relationship with a pet is like no other. By bringing animals into our homes and making them part of our families, sharing our lives with them, and caring for them, we are at our most compassionate, empathetic, and selfless. I believe that our love for animals defines our humanity.

Simply, our pets make us better people.

Now, if at that dinner party after someone asked me what I did for a living and followed up to ask how I got into this, I'd reply, "The full version of that journey is a bit too long to tell between courses." But it *is* a good story, featuring a spiteful boss, a legendary comedian, a Yorkie with unending stomach problems, a boyfriend, and a billionaire . . .

These are my tales of our pets and the City.

CHAPTER 1

How I Got Started

When I read James Herriot's classic book *All Creatures Great and Small* (now a popular, long-running PBS television show), about life as a small-town vet, it was like my internal alarm clock rang. It was time for me to change from playing make-believe veterinarian to being a real one, starting with getting a real job in a real animal hospital.

But I was only thirteen and had absolutely no idea how to get a job, much less how to become a vet.

So, I took out the family's copy of the thick Queens, New York, Yellow Pages, found the listings starting with "V," and flipped the tissue-paper-thin pages until I reached "Veterinary Hospitals." Then, I started calling each one to ask for a job. They said things like, "Call us after you have some experience" or "We can't take volunteers for insurance reasons." The worst "no" was "Call back when you grow up"—and then they hung up on me.

On my twentieth try, the vet himself answered the phone at

the Forest Hills Cat Hospital. Dr. Jay Luger listened to my teenage "I *have* to be a vet" pitch.

"I also knew I wanted to be a veterinarian when I was a kid," he said. "Why don't you come by one day after school and watch what we're doing?" I was over the moon, even just to watch, even for just one day.

Since I didn't want to arrive late, I skipped lunch so I could leave school early. Bad idea. From the moment I arrived in his office, I felt lightheaded. Whether that was from low blood sugar or excitement, I didn't know.

A smiling technician escorted me into the exam room to observe Dr. Luger's last case of the day. The patient was an old gray tabby. "This guy has lost a lot of weight recently, and I need to figure out why," he said.

He did a physical exam on the cat, and then set up to do some blood tests. Dr. Luger's assistant gently petted the patient while holding him still with his neck exposed. I leaned forward for a better look as the doctor inserted the long needle of the hypodermic syringe into the cat's jugular vein. The syringe filled with dark red blood. He transferred some of the blood into a purple-topped tube, handed it to me, and said, "Amy, turn the tube gently upside down, back and forth, so the blood doesn't clot."

As instructed, I turned the warm tube over and over and watched as the blood rushed one way and then the other. After three turns, I got a funny feeling, like my world was also flipping over . . . and then I passed out cold on the treatment room floor, just fifteen minutes after I'd walked into my first "job" at my first animal hospital.

The blood sample was saved, but my pride was not.

My hope had been to keep going to Dr. Luger's office after school every day, even though I was invited for just one. I was now too embarrassed to return at all. The next day I went back to the Yellow Pages, starting with the entry *after* Forest Hills Cat Hospital, and made more calls.

Fortunately, another vet said I could come by and observe, also for a single day. This time I made sure to eat lunch before I went.

I arrived at the hospital just as the doctor was about to begin abdominal surgery on a Labrador retriever. His assistant helped me don a cap, mask, and booties. As I entered the surgery room, I caught a glimpse of my reflection in a glass door and thought I looked very much the part of a real vet. I was extremely proud of myself.

I watched the doctor cut through the freshly shaved and prepped skin of the retriever's belly, concentrating on how sharp the scalpel must be. My breathing got increasingly louder as I inhaled and exhaled through the mask. I saw little blobs of blood bubbling up as the vet incised the skin and then cut through the belly wall, exposing the internal organs.

"This is called exploratory surgery, because I don't know the full extent of the dog's problem," the vet said to me. "So, I'm going to inspect each of his internal organs first, and then remove the mass that I know is on his liver."

I barely heard what he was saying because my breathing had now become so loud that I thought everyone else could hear it, too. And suddenly the room was blazing hot. And my vision blurred. *Why is everything black and white?* I thought just moments before I fainted to the floor. Again.

This hospital staff was very understanding, but I left that day with my tail between my legs, thoroughly embarrassed and existentially shattered. How was I ever going to become a vet if I passed out at the sight of blood?

I remained determined. I would just have to redeem myself.

And I was running out of vets in the Yellow Pages to cold call. So, the very next day (and after having lunch), I rode three city buses and showed up again—unannounced—at the first vet's cat practice.

When Dr. Luger's nurse saw me, she said dryly, "We thought you might be back. We have smelling salts ready for you." Not only did I not faint that day, I kept going back to the Forest Hills Cat Hospital for six straight years.

Fainting at the sight of blood was the first of many obstacles I've had to overcome on my path to becoming a vet.

At the end of my junior year at Barnard College, it was time to think about veterinary school applications. I needed a stellar GPA, stratospheric test scores, unreserved recommendations, and wide-ranging extracurricular experience.

The last one concerned me. By now, I knew my way around your standard house pet or lab mouse, but I had no experience with farm animals. If I could secure a summer job with a large-animal veterinary practice, then I would have a standout vet school package and be able to live my James Herriot fantasy at the same time.

From a friend of a friend, I got the name and phone number of a large-animal vet with a mobile practice in rural eastern Connecticut. This was exactly the kind of situation I was looking for.

I dialed the number and a woman answered, "Dr. Nat Johnson."

"May I speak with Dr. Johnson, please?" I asked.

"I am Dr. Johnson."

Nat as in Natalie? It had never occurred to me that this large-animal veterinarian would be a woman! Now I *had* to get a job with her. I quickly introduced myself and explained the purpose of my call, emphasizing my eagerness to learn about large animals and my willingness to do absolutely anything to be of help.

"I like your attitude, Amy," the doctor replied. "I might be able to arrange for you to spend a few weeks shadowing me. But before you decide, let me explain a few things about my practice. First of all, it is just me. I set up my equipment at the beginning of the day, drive myself to appointments, take care of my patients, and when I return at the end of the day, I wash everything and restock my truck. I work seven days a week but only a half day on Sunday."

This would be the perfect job for me. Since it would just be the two of us, I'd be able to do a lot of assisting. I would help with the washing up and stocking, too—anything to make myself useful. And it sounded just like James Herriot's practice in the Yorkshire Dales.

"I have a husband, three children, four dogs, and a cat," Dr. Johnson continued, "and we live in a house that is way too small for us. So, I'm afraid I don't have a room for you, but I do have an old horse trailer in the back. We could clean it out and put a mattress in. It doesn't have electricity or water, but you'd just be sleeping there. You would eat all your meals with us and use our bathroom facilities."

"I see," I replied. *Not exactly what I was expecting, but workable?*

"Oh, and one more thing. I run this practice on a shoestring so I'm afraid I don't have any money to pay you. But I guarantee you a wealth of experience!"

Without allowing myself to think too hard about it, I accepted Dr. Johnson's terms, and we worked out the details.

The doctor suggested I arrive on Sunday afternoon—her half day. My parents drove me to Dr. Johnson's that weekend. Passing one beautiful farm after another, we finally arrived at a ramshackle house bearing the address Dr. Johnson had given me.

I knocked on the screen door of the house. No one heard me at first above the roar of the kids yelling and dogs barking. Just as I was about to knock again, the entire family poured onto the porch to meet me. Dr. Nat introduced everyone at lightning speed, then told me to grab my duffel and follow her to the trailer out back.

A small, rusty camper sat in the center of an overgrown and untidy yard, listing slightly, its few high windows covered with years' worth of grime. I pasted on a smile, set my bag down just inside the door to the thing, and we rejoined my parents, who were eager to get back on the road for their two-hour drive home. I didn't really want to be left there, but I was determined to carry out my plan.

"You call us if you need anything," said my mother, her brow furrowed with genuine concern. She gave me a hug and kiss, which was followed by an extra-long embrace from my dad.

"Are you sure you don't want to be a people doctor like your brother?" he whispered in my ear for the hundredth time, as he smiled to hide his worry.

As promised, Dr. Nat welcomed me into the routine of her daily life and practice. Everyone rose at six, and since there was only one bathroom, we followed a strict pecking order: first Dr. Nat; then her husband, Scott; then me; and finally, the children. We ate breakfast together and then Dr. Nat and I did the dishes before setting up for rounds.

Dressed alike in tan coveralls and Wellies, the two of us went off on house calls to neighboring farms, ministering to a motley assortment of ill or pregnant cows, sheep, horses, and the occasional goat or dog. Dr. Nat hadn't been exaggerating when she said this was dirty work. Reaching our patients often necessitated slogging through mud and manure. If there was no running water at the site, I'd have to carry a brimming bucket in one hand and liquid soap and a squeeze bottle of lubricant in the other, trying hard not to spill the contents. Dr. Nat carried two heavy doctor's bags filled with equipment and medication. I couldn't imagine how much longer and harder her days were without having a helper.

When we arrived at a dairy barn, my first job was to identify the cow—usually by a red ear tag. Then I'd slip a mercury thermometer into her rectum and secure the attached clip to her tail fur so the instrument wouldn't fall to the floor or get sucked up inside her. Dr. Nat performed a complete "exterior" exam—eyes, ears, teeth, heart, lungs, limbs, mammary glands—and recited her findings as I scribbled them into her medical notebook. This was great mentoring.

Next, she instructed me to hold out my right arm and snapped a shoulder-length glove onto it. I proceeded to cleanse every inch of the cow's backside with soapy water. Then it was Dr. Nat's turn to put on a glove, lube up, and literally plunge her arm up to her shoulder into the cow's rectum. Gently, she palpated the cow's reproductive anatomy through the colon wall, describing the feel of the ovaries and size of the uterus. As I transcribed her comments, I marveled at her ability to pinpoint the status of the cow's pregnancy and predict the animal's due date. The satisfaction she got from her work was written all over her face, and I longed to possess her skills and confidence.

On a typical day, we'd repeat this process together at a minimum of three other farms. At other times, I was relegated to the role of observer, like when a horse had a laceration that needed stitching or a bull needed to be castrated. (One evening as we prepared dinner, I noticed a container in the kitchen refrigerator labeled "Bill's Bull's Balls" and I was very relieved to find that it was not on that night's menu.)

As far as I could tell, Nat's husband, Scott, had little or no interest in helping either at home or in the practice. He mainly lurked around with a beer can in his hand or lay in the front yard hammock.

Everything was fine for a couple of weeks. Then, one night as I was just dozing off in the trailer, there was a *tap-tap-tap* on the door, which, thankfully, I'd reflexively latched. I peered through the dirty window and saw Mr. Johnson swaying unsteadily on my doorstep.

Tap-tap-tap.

I stayed stone-still for ten minutes, then dared to peek through the window again.

He was gone.

I crept quietly to the door, checked the lock, and crawled back under my ratty blanket. I didn't sleep another wink that night. I'd been secretly afraid something like this might happen. From day one, he'd given me the creeps. I'd gamely convinced myself he was harmless—but deep down, I knew he was trouble. And now I had some serious thinking to do.

The next morning, I sat at breakfast, red-eyed, staring at my plate while everyone else ate their eggs. I cleaned up the dishes while Dr. Nat was feeding her beloved chickens. Scott Johnson wandered off to nap in the hammock.

Looking around to make sure nobody was nearby, I picked up the receiver of the wall phone in the kitchen and dialed my old friend and mentor, Dr. Luger, from the Forest Hills Cat Hospital. In a furtive whisper, I told him what had happened, and he didn't hesitate for a second. "However much you love the work, this is *not* what you signed up for," he said. "I'm calling your parents to pick you up."

My first impulse had been to protect my mom and dad from this sordid predicament by calling Dr. Luger, but I knew he was right, so I agreed. I went back to the trailer and threw my things into my duffel, then went off to find Dr. Nat in the coop.

"Something has come up in the City, and I-I-I have to go back," I stammered. "My parents are coming to get me."

She held my gaze for a few seconds, then nodded. She didn't ask any questions, and I didn't offer anything further, but I sensed she had an idea of what had transpired. Once again, she would be shouldering the full burden of the practice. And I'd be without a summer job.

The next morning, back in my childhood bedroom, I started the networking process all over again. My uncle had a connection. He manufactured the shipping boxes used by one of New York's largest dairy companies. He arranged for their major milk supplier to take me on as a volunteer at their farm upstate. They had plenty of room for 1,800 milking cows, but no space for a college volunteer to live, so they suggested I bring my own trailer.

Oh no, I thought. *Not another trailer.* I was desperate to follow through on my large-animal experience, so I asked my father what he thought.

"My buddy Sam has an Airstream camper, and I don't think he's been out in that thing for a decade. Let me call him and see if we can borrow it for the summer," he said.

There was no comparison between Sam's camper and the sad, rusty trailer at the Johnsons'. The Airstream had two pullout beds, a kitchen table and chairs, a fridge, and a toaster oven. Dad and I drove it far upstate, close to the Canadian border, to the farm. He again gave me his "human medicine?" look, which I ignored. And so we hugged goodbye and I began my second attempt at a large-animal summer.

As hard as I tried to earn my nonexistent salary and win everyone over with my can-do attitude, there was lingering hostility to my presence on the farm. The farmhands thought I was a spy for the dairy company, and, worse, I made the cows so nervous that milk production dropped! Word came down from the boss that I was no longer allowed to go anywhere near the milk cows. I had to figure out another way to make myself useful.

I soon did. It turns out that I was a natural at taking care of calves.

My day started at five in a small barn. First, I attended to any cows who had given birth overnight. I'd cleanse their mammary glands, massage their udders, and then strip the milk into a bucket. The first milk is called colostrum, and it contains essential life-sustaining antibodies. That was what I bottle-fed the newborn calves. It takes patience to teach the little creatures how to suckle from a bottle, and I had more of that than did the farmhands who had been doing this before I arrived at the farm. The calves bonded with me quickly, ate well, and grew faster than usual.

At eight, I took a morning break back in the Airstream, where I made myself a hearty breakfast and closed my eyes for five minutes.

Next, the really hard work began.

The farm staff relished finding tasks for me—many of which were arduous and had nothing to do with caring for animals. If nobody else wanted to do it, the chore fell on me, the volunteer from the big city. Even though I wasn't allowed in the milking barn when the cows were inside, once they were led out to pasture, it was my job to clean out the urine-and-feces-slicked gutters and other such odious and odorous undertakings.

I had never done so much intense physical labor in my life. I went from a light breakfast of granola and yogurt to wolfing down three peanut-butter-and-jelly sandwiches, and I developed arm muscles so big they tore through the cuffs on my short-sleeve shirts.

Over time, my work with the post-parturient cows made me much more comfortable with them and they with me. I was re-admitted to the milking barn, and that meant I could be present for the vet visits. My days became divided between rounds with the doctors and care and feeding of the little ones, while still doing my share of the mucking.

As much as I was now enjoying my work, I battled some fierce loneliness—particularly in the early weeks. I ate my meals alone in my trailer, and on some days exchanged not more than a few sentences of meaningful conversation with anyone. Bereft of human interaction, I did what was natural to me: I turned to animals.

A large, airy barn near my trailer was home to at least a dozen cats and kittens. I began spending my spare time there, chasing the kittens around and enjoying their company. There was one in particular—a runty little gray thing—who always seemed to be in the wrong place at the wrong time. She'd tumble from the hayloft and land on her feet, give herself a shake, and prance off to hunt mice. I named her Mieskeit, which literally means "ugly" in Yiddish, but, like all Yiddish words, it has a more nuanced connotation. I think of it as an affectionate way to call someone "funny-looking."

Mieskeit (which sounded to the farmhands like "Miss Cat") began to wait for me when I got to her barn, and she happily settled into my lap for a cuddle when I sat still long enough. Gradually, it dawned on me that she thought of herself as mine—and the feeling was mutual. She started sleeping in the trailer with me.

Slowly, I won over the human contingent as well. I knew I was "in" when the farmhands began to play practical jokes on me, one of which ended with me waist-high in manure. I laughed as loudly as anyone else at these pranks; it was worth a long hot shower to feel like one of the gang.

The summer had been all I'd hoped it would be and more. I'd amassed a wealth of knowledge and skills related to large animals, discovered I had an affinity for veterinary obstetrics (and baby animals of every kind), and made some dear friends in the process. I even got a bonus check from my notoriously frugal boss.

"You let us know if you're ever up this way," the farm owner said to me before I picked up little Mieskeit and climbed into Dad's station wagon, ready to tow Sam's camper back to the City. "And also let us know if there's anything we can do to convince those fancy schools what a good vet you're going to make."

CHAPTER 2

The Marvelous Mrs. Rivers

After graduating from veterinary school at the University of Pennsylvania, I returned to New York City to complete a grueling one-year internship at the Animal Medical Center, one of the country's premier research and teaching animal hospitals. Then I got my first real job as an associate vet at the Park East Animal Hospital. Park East was founded by a man I'll call Dr. B. It was located on the first and second floors of a limestone townhouse on East 64th Street between Park and Madison Avenues—a tony block on the Upper East Side, home to many of Manhattan's rich and powerful denizens.

Park East was different from the City's other vet hospitals. Set in a classy, cozy environment with tasteful furnishings, it was welcoming for the well-heeled clients it sought to cultivate. Park East was also the first New York City private veterinary hospital to provide twenty-four-hour nursing care for its patients. Other hospitals would close at the end of the day and leave hospitalized pets alone and unsupervised overnight. If they soiled their cage or, worse, got sick in the middle of the night, they just stayed like that until the morning, when the first staff showed up. Park East provided a very high level of care, and I was excited to be part of it.

Dr. B. was a diminutive man with a bald pate surrounded by close-cropped silver hair. He wore gold wire-rimmed glasses and was a conservative dresser in what I considered to be the Park Avenue uniform for middle-aged men: a navy blazer, dark gray slacks, Gucci loafers, a Brooks Brothers oxford cloth shirt, and Hermès tie. It was hard to tell how old he was, but I guessed anywhere from fifty to seventy. I was still in my twenties, and so anyone over forty looked old to me.

The practice was busy . . . or at least it was for Dr. B. and Dr. Gene Solomon, the senior associate. I didn't have much to do, since many clients didn't want to schedule with the new junior associate. I soon realized that the only way I could meet clients and build a following was to see them when the other vets weren't available. Love it or hate it, this meant I worked nights and weekends. My hope was that after getting to know me and my skills, clients would book a wellness exam for their pets with me in the future. And Dr. B. and Gene were only too happy to hand over their night and weekend duties.

The overnight veterinary technician was named George, three years my junior, a tall, handsome man with chiseled features and a scruffy beard. He was super smart and deeply knowledgeable about art and culture, with a photographic memory. George grew up in a fancy three-bedroom on Central Park West, and he was at ease with Park East's wealthy clients. At the time, though, he wasn't much of a people person. Nor was he a dog person. George's happy place was being surrounded by cats. He might have been a cat in a former life and so remained a nocturnal creature in this one; the overnight shift was a perfect fit for him.

I clued in very early that not all Park East clients were regarded as equal. Dr. B. designated the famous and wealthy as clients with "VIP status." All calls for VIPs were directed to Dr. B., never to the associates. It was obvious from my first days that Dr. B. was really into being a "Vet to the Stars"—and who could blame him? Clients he determined to be of lower status were automatically directed to Gene or to me. To be honest, I was happy to see *any* clients, but of course I still wanted to meet and treat some of our celebrities' pets.

Once, Yvonne, our British receptionist, called the boss's office to say, "Dr. B., Love is here." Love was an adorable bichon frise whose owner was Edmond Safra, the billionaire founder of Republic National Bank (and the first billionaire I ever met).

Dr. B. replied to Yvonne, "Is Love with the owner or the housekeeper?"

"The housekeeper."

He said, "Oh. If it's the housekeeper, she can wait."

Unbeknownst to Dr. B., that exchange was on speakerphone, and the housekeeper heard every word of it. Apparently, she did not like being disrespected, because from that day on whenever the housekeeper brought in the dog, she requested that *I* be the vet to look at Love, not Dr. B.

I knew I had to tread carefully. Being seen as the preferred vet for any of Park East's VIP clients was risky. I'd heard that in the past Dr. B. had actually fired associates if he suspected them of trying to "steal" clients and open their own practices. I'd been at Park East for a year and a half when I saw it happen firsthand. Gene had never hidden his ambition to go out on his own, plans that Dr. B. caught wind of. So one chilly winter Sunday evening, during the third quarter of the Super Bowl (when he knew Gene would never pick up his phone), Dr. B. fired him by leaving a message on his answering machine.

But I assumed I was safe at Park East; I had no intention of going anywhere, much less starting my own practice. I got along with Dr. B., and I loved my clients, their pets, and my coworkers. I was the only associate and by now a very productive part of the practice. Also, I made it clear that I wanted to stay long term. I even bought an apartment close by the hospital.

And it *was* a good practice. Most of the Park East clients were wealthy, so they could afford expensive diagnostics, procedures, and treatments that might have been too costly for others. It was a privilege to be able to use my education to make a care plan and then carry it out with no financial restrictions. Many of my colleagues at other hospitals did not have that luxury.

One Saturday around seven thirty p.m., George called me and said, "Hey, Dr. Amy. I've got one of Dr. B.'s favorite clients on the line, and she has a medical emergency with her Yorkie, Spike. She says he's pouring out bloody diarrhea."

My jaw dropped. "Holy moly," I blurted. "Spike as in *Rivers?*" I knew of only one Yorkshire terrier named Spike in the practice, and his mother was Joan Rivers. I'd been hoping to meet her since I joined Park East.

"Yup, and man, are you in for it. He's messed all over her apartment."

I have always been a huge Joan Rivers fan. As a kid, I was allowed to stay up way past bedtime to watch her when she was the super funny guest host of *The Tonight Show*. I'd heard from the Park East staff that she was incredibly gracious, but when Spike was sick, she could be impatient and might snap at you if she was dissatisfied in the slightest.

Joan was at the top of the list of Dr. B.'s VIP clients. Getting called to handle an emergency for a VIP—especially for Joan Rivers—was a big deal for me.

"George, you need to repeat her phone number. I can't read what I wrote down because I was too shaky."

He laughed. "If you're going to be like that, she's going to bite your head off."

Before I called Ms. Rivers back, I had to expend some nervous energy, so first I did a quick dance around my apartment *woo-hoo*ing (as one does in circumstances like this), and then I called my mother. She was as big a Joan Rivers fan as I was.

"Mom! Guess what? I just got an emergency call for Spike Rivers!"

No response.

"Joan Rivers's dog!" I added.

"Why are you home on a Saturday night?" asked Mom sternly.

"Joan Rivers!"

"That's fantastic, Amy," she had to admit.

My Jewish mother lived in terror that her then twenty-nine-year-old daughter would be single forever or even longer. I said goodbye, and with a pounding heart I dialed Joan Rivers.

A familiar brash voice said, "Hello?"

"Hi, Ms. Rivers, I heard Spike is sick," I said, and rapidly followed with, "You and Spike should meet me at the hospital right away."

"Who the hell are *you*?" she growled.

"Oh, sorry. I'm Dr. Amy Attas, the junior associate at Park East. I'm a vet. I did my internship at the Animal Medical Center. I got my VMD at the University of Pennsylvania—"

She didn't care about my bona fides and cut me off. "Whatever, just meet me at the hospital," she said without much humor.

We lived equidistant from the hospital, and although I moved as fast as I could, she still beat me there. She was sitting in the waiting area with Spike as I ran through the door. She looked me up and down. I couldn't help but check her out, too. Seeing her for the first time was surreal. She looked just like . . . well, like Joan Rivers, but *for real*, in 3D, breathing, right in front of me.

She wore a red dress with a fur collar, opaque stockings, black pumps with impossibly high heels, chunky gold bracelets, hanging diamond earrings, and way too many necklaces. Every inch of her was *done*, from her false eyelashes, perfect makeup, red nails that matched the dress, to her signature blond, wispy, not-a-strand-out-of-place 'do. I assumed she was going somewhere after this, perhaps Café Carlyle or a benefit at the Met. She was intimidating, dramatic, and professional. No one would ever mistake this woman for an ordinary person.

I was totally starstruck for a moment, and then I remembered my purpose. Spike was sick, I am a vet, and I needed to do my job no matter how nervous and excited I was to meet her.

"Ms. Rivers," I said, "I'm Amy . . . *Dr.* Amy Attas. Hi, Spike!"

"There's something really wrong with him," she said, clearly upset. I asked a few questions about his recent health, and she said that he had been fine and had an excellent appetite at dinner last night. Then she turned to Spike and asked him, "Didn't you love the steak from Peter Luger's?" Turning to me she added, "He loves steak."

I cringed. Rich food like steak, especially when cooked with butter like it is at the famous Brooklyn restaurant, could definitely cause GI upset. "Let's go back and I'll take a look at him," I said.

The three of us proceeded to the exam room. First, I did some quick assessment tests to determine his hydration status. I opened his mouth and touched the gums above his upper canine tooth and my finger stuck. Then I gently lifted the skin behind his neck and observed how slowly it returned to normal. He failed both tests, and blood tests later confirmed significant dehydration.

I took his temperature, and when I pulled out the rectal thermometer it was covered with "raspberry jam"—looking diarrhea. Looking up at us, he then passed a mound of loose feces containing a bunch of blood clots right on the exam table. Ms. Rivers saw the blood, and her face paled despite the makeup.

I completed the rest of my examination, and everything pointed to a diagnosis of hemorrhagic gastroenteritis, which causes severe fluid loss and makes the blood thick and sluggish and incapable of doing what it needs to do. It is eminently treatable if caught early, but patients require rehydration quickly, and the right way to do that is with intravenous fluids, meaning a hospital stay.

I explained this to Ms. Rivers, who was now getting agitated. "No. He can't stay in the hospital," she said. "He'll be distraught without me. We're partners."

"I know how difficult this will be for you both, but Spike is my concern, and I know he needs to be hospitalized to treat his dehydration quickly so he will get better."

"If you absolutely insist, but I need to know when Spike will be himself again. He's got to go on the show on Monday," she said. Spike, as it turned out, was a working dog; he regularly appeared on Joan's TV show and went onstage with her at all her appearances.

"He'll stay tonight for sure, and I'll reassess him in the morning. Now, I really need to start treating him. I'm going to take him to the treatment area where I will put in an intravenous catheter. It takes only a few minutes, and you can visit with him when I'm done."

"I want to watch," she said.

"I don't think that's a good idea," I said. "I noticed that you don't want to see anything that involves blood."

She nodded. "Okay, just tell me what you're going to do to him."

I got as far as "First, I'll shave the area on his neck where the catheter will be inserted," before she interrupted me.

"*You can't shave him!*" she yelled. "He's in Monday's show!"

"I am sorry, Ms. Rivers, it's not negotiable. The insertion area must be sterile," I explained, feeling a bit empowered saying no to her. She glowered at me as I picked up Spike and carried him into the treatment room.

Fifteen minutes later, George and I brought Spike back out to her with his catheter in place. George had covered it with a colorful bandage. She hugged Spike, gave him some red lipstick kisses, and then returned him to me while she picked up her pocketbook and coat.

"George will be with him all night," I reminded her. "You are welcome to call anytime."

"Oh, *I will*," she said. I believed her.

"Do you have any concerns?"

She opened her purse, took out her wallet, and handed George a fifty-dollar bill.

"Oh, no, Ms. Rivers!" he said, flustered. "I can't take your money."

"Take it!" she insisted. "It's my insurance policy. This way, I know you won't beat my dog." Of course, he wasn't going to beat her dog, and then I saw just the barest hint of a smile on her face. Her sense of humor could be sort of twisted. George didn't take the money.

Other than that one "joke," Joan Rivers wasn't at all funny that night. When it came to her pets, she was dead serious.

Early the next morning, Ms. Rivers and I met again at Park East. She was as hair-to-heels perfection at eight a.m. on a Sunday as she was the evening before. Spike was doing much better. His red blood cell concentration had normalized, and he was alert and hungry. He ate a jar of Gerber's baby food, a palatable and easy-to-digest meal we often give to dogs after a stomach upset. Much to my relief—and his—Spike made a semi-formed poop right in front of us, like a little gift for Mommy.

Ms. Rivers gave him a torrent of kisses and said, "I'm so glad he's doing better. We're leaving tomorrow for a show in Pittsburgh."

Pittsburgh? *Tomorrow?!* "I don't know what causes this condition, but I do know that stress can be a part of it, so it would be a good idea to let him rest a little bit longer," I said. "Traveling, eating different food, sleeping in a hotel room, going onstage with the lights, being handled by strangers, all of that stress could undo him." I know it would undo me.

"It undoes us both, but he's part of the show. He goes with me."

I gave it one last try: "I think he's well enough to go home, but I urge you to encourage him to rest."

"Are you single, Amy?" she asked, suddenly changing the subject.

"Yes, actually." Was Joan Rivers going to fix me up?

"Nice social life you have, spending Saturday night with a dog with bloody diarrhea and then back to work on Sunday morning."

No wonder my mother loved her. They were cut from the same cloth.

Over the next several months, Ms. Rivers made several more emergency visits with Spike when I was on call at night or on a weekend. It was always the same thing—vomiting and diarrhea—

but never again to the same extent as that first time. With less severe symptoms, I treated Spike with anti-nausea and diarrhea medicine and subcutaneous fluids. He perked right up each time. From this, Ms. Rivers got the idea that I had the magic touch to make him better. I knew any vet would do the same thing in that situation, but I wasn't going to tell her that.

Spike's appointment for his annual vaccines rolled around, and, instead of an assistant, Ms. Rivers herself brought him in during regular office hours and sat in the waiting room. As soon as her black pumps crossed the threshold, Yvonne called Dr. B. to tell him that his VIP client had arrived. He flew into the waiting room. "Hello, Ms. Rivers, sorry to have kept you waiting," he said. "I can see you now."

Ms. Rivers replied, "No, that's okay. I'm here to see Amy."

A pause. Then Dr. B. said, "Dr. Attas is in surgery, and she probably will be for a while."

"I'll wait."

The receptionist's head snapped up. Even the clients in neighboring chairs were suddenly paying attention. If Dr. B. thought she'd say more, he was wrong. With Spike on her lap, she started reading *People* magazine until I was available to see her.

I gave Spike his distemper vaccine and we briefly discussed his health. The visit lasted no more than fifteen minutes, less time than she'd waited for me.

Ms. Rivers left, and I went upstairs to my office to make a few calls before my next appointment. As soon as I sat down, my intercom buzzed; it was Dr. B. asking me to come to his office. He had a stern tone of voice, so I went in with trepidation. Dr. B. was seated behind his desk, I sat in the chair opposite.

He got right into it. "Amy, you need to work on your personal and professional skills."

What? At a loss, I said, "I'm sorry, did someone complain about me?"

"Just now, I was talking to Ms. Rivers, and she called you 'Amy.' She didn't call you 'Dr. Attas.' That's a sign she doesn't respect you."

I blinked, confused. "She waited for me to take care of her dog, which I think shows a great deal of respect," I said. "And she understands that I have a first name, and that it's okay to call me by it."

He glared at me. "You need to work harder on your skills," he repeated, digging in, and looking down, returned to his paperwork. I left the room.

I tried to shake off that exchange, but it was just so weird. I went back downstairs to greet my next patient and mentioned to Yvonne what just happened. "I'm not surprised," she said. "When Ms. Rivers said she'd rather wait for you than see him, smoke came out of his ears."

Lesson: Never underestimate a boss's wounded ego.

From that day forward, Dr. B. paid very close attention to which VIP clients asked for me. I didn't set out to win over any of his clients, but as I got to know them during off-hours emergency visits, many did start to request me for their regular checkups. I kept my head down and just did my job.

I must have been doing it well because after just three years of working there, Dr. B. asked me, "Amy, how would you feel about becoming my partner?"

Well, I was shocked and flattered and immediately saw dollar signs floating in my eyes. My salary was just $40,000. If you haven't heard, living in New York is expensive. I had student loans and now a mortgage. Any bump in income would have made a huge difference for me. Surely, a partner at Park East would earn a lot more than $40,000.

As if reading my mind, he said, "The practice doesn't make a profit so I can't give you a raise, but I will put your name above the line on our stationery."

Considering the volume of cases that came through the doors—between Dr. B., our new associate Dr. Rick Baum, and me—we saw dozens of patients in a day, and so I had just assumed Park East was profitable. It didn't matter. I loved working here and I was honored to be asked to be a partner.

After a delay of many weeks, Dr. B. gave me some paperwork to sign. Looking forward to a partnership agreement, I saw instead the words "Restrictive Covenant." It was a non-compete agreement. The document stated that I couldn't practice veterinary medicine anywhere in New York City for a year if I left Park East for any reason, which could include *terminating me without cause*. I didn't go to that school (law), but this didn't sound like a good way to start a partnership.

I called my former vet school professor James Wilson, an expert in this area, who told me, "This is so extreme, Amy, no judge would ever uphold this, but it would cost you a lot of money fighting him over it in court if it ever came to this." I didn't sign it.

In the summer of 1992, a year or so after the partnership and subsequent discussions about selling me the practice, Dr. B. asked me, "Amy, can you leave next Wednesday evening open?" That date was August 5, my four-year anniversary of working at Park East. "I'd like to take you to dinner, and we can discuss a bonus and a raise since you had a good year."

Finally.

"That sounds great!" I blurted. I knew I was right to stick it out.

"I made us a reservation at Orso," he said, smiling. Dr. B. knew it was my favorite restaurant. I was excited about this dinner, not only for Orso's paper-thin garlic pizza bread but also because it was appropriately named after the owner's beloved dog. It seemed like an auspicious sign that I was finally going to get a much-needed raise.

Around five p.m., Dr. B. called me into his office.

Maybe he was going to give me a cash bonus before *dinner?*

He said, "Given the fact that it's your work anniversary, I thought it would be a good idea for us to have a review. Why don't you start?"

Something in my gut told me not to. I said, "No, please, you're the boss. I think that you should start."

He said, "Amy, I don't think that you have the kind of personality that I want to go forward with into the next decade. You need to take all of your personal belongings and leave now. And don't come back to this practice again."

Did he really just say that?

I left his office, went into mine, dumped my things into a bag, walked downstairs to the X-ray room where I picked up my blind pug Bumper, who always came to work with me, and exited the building. No tears, just numb shock.

With my dog under one arm and a bulging bag on my shoulder, I zombie-walked to my boyfriend Steve's office at 57th Street and Sixth Avenue. (Yes, Mom, I finally had a boyfriend—one who would eventually become my husband.) He looked at me and said to the person he was on the phone with, "I have to hang up. Amy just walked in. I think she's been fired."

Gene had tried to warn me. The partnership talk was fake, as was the subsequent tease to sell me the practice, both just stalling tactics. I was fired on Wednesday evening, and the vet he'd already hired to replace me was sitting at my desk on Thursday morning.

That first night after I was dismissed, when the shock and numbness wore off, I veered between livid and terrified. When clients heard that I'd been summarily fired, they might think I deserved it. *Did Amy kill someone's dog? Is she on drugs? Did she steal?* My reputation was all I had, and it seemed to me that he fired me abruptly precisely to damage it.

"Where am I going to work? What am I going to do?" I asked both myself and Steve over and over as we sat up all night thinking and talking. Over the last few years, I'd been solicited by other veterinarians to join their practices. But I wasn't so keen to rush into a similar role, working for another entitled middle-aged man, where the same thing could happen again.

At eight the next morning, two clients called me at home. One was the author Isabelle Holland, whose cat, Peter, had been my patient for all four years at Park East. Elderly, with advanced kidney disease, Peter was scheduled to be euthanized. When she called the hospital to confirm the appointment and heard I was no longer working there without further information, she canceled and tracked me down. "No one knows Peter like you do. And you are so sweet with him. I want *you* to put Peter to sleep," she said, and I started to cry.

The other message was from my client whose West Highland white terrier, Chutney, had lymphoma and was scheduled for chemotherapy that day. She echoed Isabelle's sentiment, that she wanted only me to treat her beloved pet.

The next call I received was from George, the overnight tech. He said simply, "I heard. How can I help you?"

"Can you come with me on two house calls today?" If I was going to treat my patients at home, I would need another set of trained hands. George agreed with not one second of hesitation.

I didn't have time to bask in gratitude for the loyalty and kindness of my coworker and clients. I focused on the practical. I called Gene and told him that Dr. B. had given me the axe. "Welcome to the club," he said. "I'll skip the 'I told you so.' My hospital is your hospital. Come by for whatever you need, and we'll figure everything out when your world stops spinning."

The first thing Gene did when I arrived at his practice, the Center for Veterinary Care, was hand me the elegant leather house call bag I had given to him as a farewell gift when he left Park East two years earlier. That gesture made me cry, too.

"Stop," he said. "Load the bag."

I composed myself and loaded it full of the supplies and medications I would need and was off and running—cabbing, actually—to my two appointments of the day.

The next day, I made *four* house calls. And the day after that, four more. George was happy to work part-time with me secretly during the day and put in his overnight hours at Park East. The word was getting out, and I had more calls every day.

I realized that I might be able to just keep doing house calls and not have to work at a clinic or hospital for anyone else ever again. I could be in charge of my destiny, a prospect that was far more exciting than going into massive debt to buy someone else's practice.

I asked Steve, "Do you think there might be something here? A house call practice?"

"I don't know if it's economically possible, but I do know you'd be a superstar at it. It's a perfect fit for your very personal style of practice," he said.

He was the only one who believed I could do it. I asked several other trusted advisers. Some said, "It's a novelty. People will get tired of it." Others warned of parking tickets and hemorrhoids from spending so much time in a car. The consensus was to go ahead and do house calls "until you figure out where you land."

I had no idea how to execute what I was envisioning. Some vets visited patients at home after regular hospital hours, but I'd never heard of a full-time Manhattan house call–exclusive practice. There had been one or two vets in the City doing it ad hoc, but they gave it up and went back to a hospital setting.

I knew it could work. Clients might even prefer the vet to treat their pets where they all felt most comfortable. If I had a steady source for medications and equipment, a place to store them, and access to Gene's hospital for surgeries, I thought I could pull this off. I just needed clients.

I placed advertisements in *The New York Times*, *New York* magazine, and *The New Yorker*, as well as in the local Upper East and West Side newspapers and giveaways, that read simply, "Dr. Amy Attas, formerly of Park East Animal Hospital, is now available for veterinary house calls in the comfort of your own home."

Next, I called an even bigger bullhorn to get the word out, in fact the biggest I knew. Joan Rivers answered my phone call on two rings. "Hello, Ms. Rivers," I said. "I just wanted you to know that I've left Park East and am now available for house calls."

"What happened?" she asked.

"Do you want the long story or the short version?"

"I want *every single detail,* and I promise you everybody on the Upper East Side is going to know every detail, too."

So I told her the long version, going back some three years to the day when she told Dr. B. that she'd rather wait for me to finish a surgery than work with him. That planted the seed in his mind that I might be a threat to him. "So, in a way," I told her, "*you* got me fired."

She laughed her classic, throaty laugh and said, "Don't worry, I'll make it up to you."

She sure did. The woman with the famous catchphrase "Can we talk?" called everyone she knew and told them about my new practice. She single-handedly drummed up word-of-mouth buzz and became not only one of my most loyal clients but also, as it evolved over the decades, a dear friend.

CHAPTER 3

My Agility Training

In the earliest days of my new house call practice, City Pets, I had to learn a whole new set of skills requiring adaptability and flexibility. Now I had to run a business. I had to advertise, find clients, satisfy them, hire and manage staff, send bills, pay bills—and all the unforeseen but critical tasks that one needs to get started and become successful.

My parents got involved, generating reminder postcards to send my new clients when their pets were due for vaccines. Dad would read their information aloud because his handwriting was illegible, and Mom would write the cards. They even handed out fliers at events. Along with my boyfriend Steve, they were my biggest cheerleaders—but even though my new business seemed promising, I soon realized that I had a lot to learn.

I felt like I was doing the training that competitive dogs go through. I had to develop the ability—the *agility*—to jump higher, speed up, slow down, and suddenly change direction to keep moving forward. My eyes had to dart and be sharp, ears perked up, and even my sixth sense had to be on high alert to make this people-facing business successful. Particularly Manhattan people. Especially Manhattan *animal* people.

It was my first appointment in the first full week of my reinvented career. I arrived at an Upper East Side townhouse (meaning: wealthy), where I was scheduled to see Rocky. Rocky was an eleven-year-old massive, occasionally aggressive, unneutered male rottweiler who had a painful swollen eye. He belonged to Robert Chapin, a successful businessman who owned real estate all around Manhattan as well as several Michelin-starred restaurants. After those restaurants, Rocky was his true love.

I met them both at Park East when Dr. B. surprisingly transferred Rocky's appointment to me. I say surprisingly, because Mr. Chapin was one of his VIP clients. I understood why I got the appointment only after the exam ended and Mr. Chapin told me that I was the first veterinarian Rocky hadn't bitten.

Visiting them at home for the first time, I marveled at what looked like a perfect Mayfair townhouse, and I was excited to see if the inside was as impressive as the outside.

I rang the bell. A butler in white tie and gloves opened the door.

"I'm Dr. Amy Attas, the vet," I said, trying to see inside over his shoulder. "I have an appointment to see Rocky." The butler shouldered some of my equipment bags—which I'd schlepped myself in a cab that morning—and ushered me in.

As soon as you enter someone's personal space, you learn so much about them. Right off the bat, I saw that Mr. Chapin was a man living in the wrong era. While I would soon see that all the Upper East Side homes were decorated either in a modern, sleek minimalist style or with Buatta-like explosions of floral chintz everywhere, this home was old Europe. It felt like an English country estate: a regal clutter of red-leather Chesterfield couches, ornate Georgian furniture with clawed feet, overlapping Oriental rugs, and dark wood paneling. On every surface were carved lamps, obviously expensive glassware, and hung portraits.

"Right in here," said the butler, showing me into the dining room though a pair of floor-to-twelve-foot-ceiling French doors with beveled glass panels that might have been as old as the house itself. A uniformed maid was just finishing, and the room smelled like old wood and lemon Pledge. Around the polished mahogany table sat sixteen Queen Anne chairs. The Georgian sideboard was laden with a gleaming antique silver tea service that I could picture a Downton Abbey butler furiously polishing nightly (my father was a silversmith so I knew enough to be impressed).

I was marveling at the trip back in time when the butler returned me back to the present. "Mr. Chapin will be with you in ten minutes," he announced. He left, drawing the glass-paneled doors closed behind him.

It took all of five minutes for me to set up the equipment on the dining table. I thought I had enough time to duck into the nearby bathroom. I opened the double doors and called out, "I'll just be in the powder room." No one responded.

When I returned, Mr. Chapin was still nowhere in sight. But, on the other side of the table, I spotted Rocky and went in. His left eye was indeed swollen shut. The right eye focused on me, and it was not happy.

In a heartbeat Rocky lunged toward me, baring large teeth, and emitted a deep growl that was more like a roar. Instinct took over. I ran out of the room, grabbed the knobs of the double doors, and slammed them shut just a millisecond before Rocky crashed into them so hard I thought the glass panels would shatter.

Shaking, I held the doors closed with all my strength while Rocky body-slammed them, snarling and barking his head off, drool splattering the glass. If I'd been a split-second slower or he'd seen me sooner, there was no doubt I would have been injured. His altered vision from that swollen left eye probably saved me.

The sound of Rocky's attack made the butler, maid, and Mr. Chapin all come running, and each apologized profusely. My heart pounding, I said, "I'm fine. It was my fault. I shouldn't have gone in there without you."

I was smarter than this and mad at myself. I knew that Rocky had the potential to be aggressive and it was I who had just committed an aggressive act by entering his territory. It's possible that I wasn't paying 100 percent attention when I walked in, being so taken by the interior décor. I should have waited for Mr. Chapin before I went in.

He said, "I'm so sorry, sweetie. Are you okay? You're shaken up. We'll reschedule."

I pulled myself together. "No," I said. "Rocky's in pain. I'll treat him now." I needed to see this through. If I showed up at a client's home to treat a pet, I was going to do it, no matter what I encountered on the other side of the door.

"So what now?" he asked, as I recovered from the attack and we both stared at Rocky through the glass doors. The enormous dog had finally stopped crashing against them. He was now sitting but still glaring at me through his one good eye.

"Go in first and leash him," I directed.

While the butler and maid cowered behind me in the hallway, Mr. Chapin went into the dining room, closed the doors, and spoke softly to his pet. At eleven, though Rocky was a senior rottweiler and had already outlived his breed's typical life span, he hadn't slowed down.

Once Rocky was leashed and seated next to Mr. Chapin, I went in. On rubbery legs, I nonetheless tried to appear calm and confident for all our sakes. "Let's have a look at that eye," I said to Rocky in a let's-make-up-and-stay-friends voice.

My equipment was in place on the table, so I gloved up and bent down to go eye-to-eye with the beast that had just tried to tear my head off. I began in a soft, calm voice to explain to both my client and my patient what I was about to do.

"I'm going to hold your eyelid open with my fingers and then touch this strip of paper to your eyeball for thirty seconds to check for dry eye." The strip of filter paper was marked in millimeters to measure quantity and quality of tear production. Dogs, like people, can get acutely dry eyes, which hurts. Rocky might have a corneal ulcer, a wickedly painful condition where the surface layer of cells is damaged or missing, which I believed to be the problem. A damaged cornea might also explain Rocky's supercharged aggressive behavior. But first I had to rule out dry eye, and to do that, I had to put my nose within a few inches of his massive teeth.

"Good boy," I said soothingly while doing the test. Meanwhile, I was trying to remember to breathe.

Rocky was probably tired from battering himself against the doors because he submitted to the filter test without snapping or snarling. His tear production was normal.

"Now I'm going to put a few drops of topical anesthesia in your eye," I said. "You'll feel much better." Once the drops were in, Rocky wouldn't feel pain for twenty minutes. Instantly his shoulders relaxed. I got the sense that he went from being eager to kill me to being only mildly interested in my death.

Quickly, before the anesthetic could wear off, I held his lid open with one hand and instilled a drop of orange stain to check the integrity of the cornea, the top layer of the eye. Part of it glowed fluorescent green. Bingo.

"No wonder you're in a mood," I said. "You've got a large corneal ulcer."

"Will he go blind?" asked Mr. Chapin.

"No, he won't, and I am starting his treatment right now."

I gave him an extra dose of topical anesthetic and then applied the first dose of medication to heal the ulcer. Rocky was already feeling better because of the anesthetic, and when I finished, he lay down on the Oriental rug and wagged his nub of a tail. I'm not saying he was suddenly weak and helpless, but in this scenario, Rocky was like the lion with a thorn just pulled from his foot, which of course made me the mouse.

All done, I packed up my equipment, my heartbeat finally returning to normal. Mr. Chapin even helped me carry my bags to the front door. "That wasn't so bad, was it?" he said, ever the downplayer.

I nodded but said, "It could have been worse."

"See you in a few months for Rocky's boosters?" he asked. "We'll be on our best behavior, I promise."

"Of course," I said. Until then, I had a rule never to use tranquilizers for exams, but after that appointment, I thought I might make an exception . . . but not for Rocky. For me!

From that day on, I've never entered the territory of an aggressive dog, even one who knows me. Instead, I make sure I am the first in the room and let the dog come to me.

This time, though I'd almost been mauled, I chalked it up as a win. All week long, I'd been worried about every aspect of trying to start a house call practice. I was afraid I'd fail, that I didn't know what I was doing, that it was impossible to treat patients without a nurse, that clients wouldn't want me caring for their pets at home—that I wouldn't even *have* clients.

But one thing I had not anticipated was a violent attack from a patient. I had every reason to be scared, but now that it was over, I felt a rush of confidence. I hadn't given up. I'd faced the angry animal and treated him—and I did it all right in front of the client. Both man and beast were grateful.

There was no time to bask in glory, though. I flagged down a taxi, piled my stuff inside, and gave the cabdriver the address of the next appointment. I knew I would figure it all out eventually. *One down, a lifetime to go.*

Getting around Manhattan is like running an obstacle course, weaving through traffic and working garbage trucks, unanticipated street closures, jaywalkers, potholes and randomly uncovered manholes, rush hours and school buses. Rainstorms are my worst enemy. One drop and the sidewalks of Manhattan are suddenly clogged with slow, umbrella-wielding pedestrians, making it a huge pain to wheel my equipment suitcase around. Worse, with just a touch of snow, New Yorkers outright forget how to drive, and with a little more snow, side streets shrink to one lane hemmed in by unclimbable snowbanks, and remarkably deep pools of dirty slush appear on each corner.

I tried taking the subway to get from house call to house call, but hauling my equipment up and down those stairs ten times a day was unworkable. I was stuck taking taxis. Back then (and now), New York City cabs were hit or miss in terms of cleanliness and comfort. Some had no suspension, others sticky, duct-taped seats, and almost all had the last passenger's trash on the floor and nauseating "air fresheners" dangling from the mirror. Sitting in the back of a lurching cab for hours each day was making me sick. Literally.

At the end of a particularly trying day, I returned home and said to Steve, "I've had a premonition. I am going to die in the back seat of a taxi or be murdered by someone trying to steal one from me."

Steve, ever the problem solver, said simply, "Hire a driver."

"Are you crazy? I can't afford a driver."

He took one look at me, drenched and miserable from the day's travails, and said, "You can't afford not to. And hire an administrative assistant, too."

I placed an ad for a driver in *Pennysaver*, a thin local giveaway rag, and that brought me a young man, around twenty, named Burt. Burt drove down from Harlem for an interview at Steve's office, where I'd set up my base of operations in a corner of his conference room.

Burt was handsome and well-dressed in a blue blazer, Gucci loafers, and carrying a Louis Vuitton briefcase, all for an interview to be my driver. After we chatted, I said, "Drive me around the neighborhood. Show me what you got."

"Great," he said, eagerly. "My BMW is parked downstairs. I snagged a great spot right out front."

Oh, dear. Right out front? There were no legal parking spots on 57th Street, and we'd been talking for half an hour already. "We'd better hurry," I said, not wanting to scare him.

We went outside and found the street empty where his car was once parked, right under a large sign that read NO PARKING ANY-TIME. TOW-AWAY ZONE.

Poor Burt said sheepishly, "How did I miss that?"

He looked so distraught that I did the only thing I could think of. I hired him. I told him to retrieve his car from the City's impound lot and come to work the next day.

Burt was a nice guy and a good driver, and he became an essential part of our team. He whisked me and George, now my regular vet tech, around from house call to house call. What a dream! I had to admit to Steve that this made my job so much easier, and I was able to book more appointments as a result.

In fact, things were going so well, I took my first weekend off in four months and went to visit my parents in Florida. Burt drove Steve and me to the airport one Friday after work, and I gave him my flight information so he could pick us up when we returned on Sunday evening.

As soon as the plane landed at LaGuardia Airport on Sunday, my beeper (pre-cell phone days) began going off nonstop. It was Burt's number. I rushed off the plane and frantically looked for a pay phone so I could call him back.

"What are you so upset about?" Steve asked.

"It's Burt. I have a bad feeling about this."

"Come on, it's not like he's in jail or anything."

I dialed the number and a woman answered. It was Burt's mom. She was calling to tell me that Burt was in jail.

"And so he can't pick you up tonight or tomorrow morning," she said, "but don't worry. His best friend Corey is going to pick you up Monday morning at the usual spot."

Corey also had a new BMW and a great attitude, but he told me right away that he'd been on a waiting list for three years to work for the NYC Parks Department. Two months after I hired him, he got the call he'd been hoping for and left me to work for the City. Corey handed me off to *his* best friend, Anthony, a shy young man over six feet tall. Anthony was so tall he had to push the driver's seat so far back in his BMW that there was no room for anyone behind him, even for a short person like me. But we made it work.

Anthony did have one flaw. Occasionally, while we were upstairs in an apartment seeing a patient, he would tilt the seat way back and fall asleep. Once I came back to the car and found him sleeping so deeply he didn't even know he'd gotten a ticket.

"Anthony, don't sleep between calls. I can't afford the tickets!" I exclaimed, knowing I'd have to pay them.

"Sorry, Dr. Amy. It just gets so boring waiting. And with the sun streaming in my eyes they just start to close."

It was true we didn't have a lot of business in those early years, and my driver wasn't yet tasked with pickups and drop-offs all around town while the team was upstairs doing its work. "Why don't you keep yourself busy while I'm upstairs? Read a book or something," I suggested.

"Books are boring."

"*Boring* books are boring," I retorted. "Read about things that interest you."

I recalled some weeks ago he said he saw the film *Malcom X*, and so the next day I brought him a copy of *The Autobiography of Malcolm X*. He looked at it skeptically but reluctantly promised he would read at least the first chapter.

Later that same day, we were behind schedule, and I rushed back to the car ready to go to a client who was angry we were late. George and I loaded our equipment quickly and jumped in the car. But Anthony didn't start the engine. *Asleep again?!*

"Anthony! What's the matter?! We have to go. I'm really late!"

"Just a minute, Dr. A. I have only two more pages in this chapter."

I was floored. That was worth being late for. Anthony never slept in the car again, but he did get through a slew of books during business hours.

❧

Now that my driver issue was settled and George had committed to being my vet tech (the first of several excellent nurses I've worked with over the years; Shari, Carida, and Jeanine come later), I had to find an assistant. By now I had taken over the whole conference room in Steve's office to store my equipment, supplies, and records. For the time being, it was my office.

My client Rachel was a headhunter who found jobs for actresses who were between acting gigs, and through her I hired some talented, lovely women. But as soon as I got one trained, she was invariably cast in an out-of-town production of *Oklahoma!* or got recurring parts on *Law & Order* and had to quit. Happy for them, but their big breaks left me high and dry.

So actresses were out, and instead Rachel sent me Radio City Rockettes. Greta, twenty-two, from Wisconsin, was friendly, hardworking, and gorgeous beyond belief with mile-long legs. She manned the conference room office while I went out on rounds, and Steve was just fine with that.

Greta took the call from a new client on East 96th Street. Brenda Collins was moving to California and taking her four cats with her. They all needed vaccinations and travel certificates. Seeing four pets in one location, plus the vaccinations and travel certificates, would make this a lucrative visit.

One by one, I did the exam and vaccinations for the first three cats.

The fourth cat, Precious, was obviously nervous. (Why do the difficult patients always have sweet names like *Precious*?) I got him from his hiding place myself and gently carried him back to where my equipment was set up. Brenda reached toward Precious to comfort him. I could tell from the tension in his body that

Precious was going to bite her, so without thinking, with my right hand I pushed Brenda safely back, keeping Precious in my left. In a flash, he sunk his teeth deep into my right wrist and held on.

Owww! That truly hurt.

Carefully and calmly, George extricated the cat from my flesh with a heavy towel around the cat. My hand immediately began to swell. Blinking away tears, I ignored the pain, completed the exam, and administered the vaccines Precious needed for travel.

When we got to the car, Anthony saw my face and said, "Dr. Amy, are you okay?"

I said, "Change of plans," and gave him the address of my doctor.

George usually sat up front, but now he squished into the back seat with me. He examined my rapidly swelling and darkening hand and said, "Anthony, step on it!" He knew full well how dangerous cat bites can be. He had five cats himself.

I wound up visiting three doctors, including my brother Lewis, a quadruple-boarded physician in New Jersey. In the end, a hand surgeon in Manhattan said that I'd need to check into the hospital and get three weeks of a constant 24/7 IV antibiotic drip. I couldn't do that! I had a new practice to run.

"It's that or you could lose your hand," she said.

That did sound bad.

I asked the doctor, "Can I arrange for me to get my IV treatment *at home?*" I knew that was possible because some of my brother's cancer patients got their IV drugs at home.

She glared at me and said, "What is this? *Medicine by negotiation?*"

It was, and I insisted. Later that day a nurse came to my apartment and placed an intravenous catheter in my left arm. Steve and George set up a schedule to change the IV drip bag three times each day. During one of his visits, George joked that he would inject an air bubble if I didn't give him a raise. Of course, I promised the raise.

I was utterly miserable for the entire three weeks, even though I loved the irony of the house call doctor getting her own treatment at home. I had so much to do both professionally and personally, and now I couldn't even feed myself.

Worse still, Steve and I were having our engagement party (!) in just six weeks, and I hadn't had time to buy a dress before the cat bite. I made a call to the boutique one block away from my apartment, and three hours later two clothing racks filled with beautiful party dresses were wheeled down the sidewalk from the store. The boutique owner told me to hold on to anything I liked, and I could try them on when I was feeling better; they'd pick up the rest. It was an act of total kindness. Eventually, I bought *two* dresses, one for the party and one just to make me feel better.

It took the full three weeks of antibiotics until I was deemed well enough to go back to work. I eased back into appointments, but because of lingering pain, I couldn't do surgery for a while and I referred those cases to surgical specialists. When I was ready, I scheduled my first surgery at the Center for Veterinary Care, Gene's hospital.

My patient that day, a small dog, had a retained testicle that hadn't descended into the scrotal sac and was still in his belly. He was scheduled to be neutered, which in his case meant removing the scrotal testicle and then going into the abdomen to take out the one that had not descended. It was a simple surgery that I'd done many times before.

I made the initial incision in the abdomen and started hunting around for the testicle. After five minutes, I still couldn't locate it.

Obviously it had to be in there. My forehead beaded with sweat, and the idea formed in my mind that I was never going to find the testicle and this surgery would never end. My head pounded.

I was in the midst of a panic attack. My first. I knew that my anxiety was irrational and wouldn't last, but that didn't lessen it one bit. I had a patient under anesthesia, and I wasn't performing my job.

"Get Gene," I said to the nurse assisting me. "Hurry!"

Gene rushed into the OR. "What's the matter?"

"I can't do this," I said. "You have to take over."

He saw instantly that I was in the grip of anxiety, but he said, "I'm not going to scrub in. You're going to finish this. Take a breath. Tell me, what are you doing?"

"I'm looking for the testicle," I replied.

"Where should it be? Okay, good, now go there."

A few more minutes of searching, and I found it. I nearly burst into tears with relief.

"What are you going to do now?" he asked.

"I'm going to remove it."

Gene stayed and talked me through the whole procedure, step by step. With his patience, I finished the surgery and the dog was 100 percent fine.

But I wasn't. I sat in the break room and shook for a solid hour afterward.

Gene said, "I told you that you could do it."

"You're right. I did it. But it's the last surgery I'm ever going to do."

And it was. Having a panic attack with someone's dog under anesthesia was one of the worst experiences of my life as a vet. I have the greatest respect for my colleagues who are board certified in surgery and henceforth would happily refer my patients to the very best among them.

I hit a big mental obstacle during that surgery. I didn't try to get over it, go through it, or duck under it. I just turned around. One of the greatest agility skills you can master is self-awareness, knowing when to stop, assess, and even change direction from a wrong path to one that is better for you. And in truth, this pivot—not to do my own surgeries but to refer them to board-certified surgeons—has proven to be a blessing in disguise. I prefer patients who are awake and wagging their tails or purring.

CHAPTER 4

A Bond Like No Other

Rumor has it that my first word was "puppy." That was a little odd since my family didn't even have a dog when I was that young. But from that early age I knew I loved dogs—all animals, in fact— and I had to have one.

My brother Lew, our dad, and I were all in cahoots on this. The holdout was Mom, who was afraid of dogs. She also had her hands full taking care of the family and working at Dad's factory, Paramount Silversmiths, as the bookkeeper. And Mom knew that despite what we promised, if we did get a dog all the responsibilities would fall on her. But we kept trying.

Dad loved the dogs with pushed-in faces and eventually got Mom to agree to look at both a boxer and a bulldog. First, they visited a boxer breeder. When the large dogs came running out of the house, Mom wouldn't even get out of the car! Too scary. A similar thing happened the next week at a bulldog breeder. Mom just said a flat out *"No!"* to them, too.

Dad had a third choice in his back pocket: pugs. Pugs are a lot smaller than both boxers and bulldogs, and their pushed-in faces are full of expression. Back in the early 1960s, pugs weren't at all popular, and most people—including Mom—had never even seen one. Dad had done his research and found a breeder a few hours away. Mom agreed to one final try. (There may have been a promise of an Oldsmobile Cutlass Supreme involved, but I can't verify that.)

The next Saturday, my grandparents came to take care of me and Lew while my parents left for the daylong trip to the pug breeder. There they found Duchess, a three-year-old female pug who'd had a few litters already and was now up for adoption. Sweet-natured, Duchess had a black muzzle, quarter-sized dark chocolate eyes, jet black ears that I swear were made of velvet, a cute fawn-colored body, and a tail shaped like a cheese Danish.

"I think I could manage to live with this dog," said Mom reluctantly, and that was all Dad needed to hear. He didn't wait for her second thoughts but agreed to adopt Duchess immediately. Although I never asked, I think he really wanted a pug all along and had set Mom up by taking her to see the bigger dogs first.

Duchess sat on Mom's lap in the car on the way home. Both were awkward and nervous—and then Duchess pooped on Mom's dress. "That means she loves you," said Dad hopefully.

"Just drive," said Mom.

Lew and I adored Duchess on sight, and she was instantly a part of the family. She came everywhere with us.

Sometimes, people would stop us on the street and say, "That is the *ugliest* dog I've ever seen," and Dad had a standard response: "You wish you were as beautiful in *your* species as she is in hers!" Some would say to him, "You know, you and your dog look exactly alike." They weren't wrong. My father *did* look like a pug, which may be why he was attracted to the squished-face breeds.

Duchess became my best friend. I occasionally dressed her up in baby onesies and wheeled her around in a carriage, but that didn't seem to put her off. And one time I shared so many of my Swedish fish candies with her that she pooped green, red, yellow, and orange for the next three days. I even entered Duchess in our elementary school talent show. Her talent? She could shell a sunflower seed in her mouth: crack it open, drop the shell on the floor, and then eat just the seed. Not a great audience visual but at least better than the collie who defecated onstage.

I shared everything about my life with Duchess. When I whispered my secrets into her velvet ears, she would stare back at me with deep, soulful eyes like she really understood. Later, in adolescence, when I cried over some stupid boy or mean-girl drama, Duchess licked away my tears. She provided a place of comfort and security for me, and I learned from her what a unique and special bond two species can have with each other.

One amazing human–pet relationship that still takes my breath away was between Butter, a golden retriever, and Ellen Burstein, once a muckraking TV journalist and author. Ellen was diagnosed with multiple sclerosis fifteen years before I met her. She'd recently moved back to New York for cutting-edge MS treatment, and her twin sister, Patricia, and another sister, Karen, a judge who would later run for attorney general of New York State, were both living in New York City.

I didn't know anything about Ellen when I arrived for that first appointment. All I knew was that I was going to meet a new client for a wellness check on her neutered ten-year-old male golden.

Ellen lived in a modest two-bedroom apartment in a modern building on Columbus Avenue. When I entered the lobby, the doorman waved me to the elevator and said, "Go on up. Ellen has been waiting for you."

I hadn't even had a chance to say that I was the vet!

I rang the doorbell. Silence. I immediately looked down at my paperwork to confirm I was at the right apartment because normally my dog patients start barking when I approach the front door, sometimes even before I touch the doorbell. But a ten-year-old golden not barking? *Maybe he's already lost his sense of hearing?*

I was preparing my thoughts for a senior dog exam, and just as I was about to ring again, I heard a faint, "Just a minute . . ." The door slowly opened, but I saw no one on the other side. I scanned around for about a millisecond and eventually noticed Butter, down at dog height. My patient was standing inside the door, wagging his tail as he dropped from his mouth the pully that enabled him to open the handle of the front door with his mouth. *That's a first.*

I said, "Hello, Butter."

From somewhere inside, Ellen called out, "I'm in here. Butter will show you."

Butter invited me inside with the tilt of his head, and then nudged the door closed behind us. Thoroughly impressed with his training, I followed him down the hallway with my wheelie suitcase full of equipment. Ellen was sitting in a wheelchair in a sparsely furnished living room. A mid-fortyish-year-old woman with close-cropped brown hair, she smiled when she said, "I see you've met Butter. He's my best friend, confidant, twenty-four-hour caretaker, and the most wonderful dog that ever was!"

I smiled back and tried not to stare at Ellen, who was in an awkward position in her wheelchair. It was obvious that she had a significant disability, and I was sure there must be a caregiver somewhere in the apartment who would get her sorted out.

I sat near her and began to ask some background questions about Butter. We went over what he ate, his bathroom habits, his prior medical conditions, and his vaccine history. While we were talking, Butter put his head on her lap and adjusted his body so his front left leg lay across her legs.

"What a sweet show of affection," I commented.

"He's just doing his job. Sometimes I have uncontrollable jerking motions, which could make me fall out of my wheelchair. His leg across me keeps me from falling. He does something similar at night. He sleeps completely across my body to make sure I don't fall out of bed," she said. "That used to happen before he came into my life."

Nobody taught Butter to do this. He seemed to know what Ellen needed, and he just did it. She went on to describe herself as fiercely independent and said she couldn't handle having people around her all day even though she needed care. But if Butter was with her, she could be alone for hours without fear of hurting herself.

I was ready to start the exam and called Butter over to me. He gently nudged Ellen as if to ask if he could leave her and go to me, and I saw the very slightest nod of her head. As he walked the ten feet to where I was waiting, I asked Ellen if there was anything she was concerned about.

"He seems fine, but I want you two to establish a relationship now while he is healthy. He's getting older and I'm worried that I might miss something important about his health. If it's not a problem, I want to schedule frequent wellness exams," she continued. "Butter is my life."

"Of course, that will be my pleasure," I replied. Ellen watched as I examined every inch of Butter while I spoke a running commentary on how good he looked. She watched intently until I took the syringe and tubes out to take his blood.

"You know, I have my blood taken all the time and I always look," she said. "But I can't with Butter." She turned her head slightly away. Moving her neck and her arms slightly were the only movements available to her.

"I'll let you know tomorrow what the lab results are," I said when I finished. "But from my exam today, aside from wax in his ears and some dental tartar, I am pleased to tell you that you've got a healthy dog here."

"Thank you for making me smile. I look forward to your call tomorrow. It's best to ring in the afternoon when Kathy is here to help me. Now, Butter, can you get my purse?" she asked him. To me she asked, "How much do I owe you?"

I explained my invoice while Butter went to a nearby chair and picked up the handle of her pocketbook. He walked over to me with it dangling from his mouth. Ellen asked, "Would you mind? My checkbook is inside. Go ahead and fill in the amount, and I'll sign it."

I wrote the check, tore it from her checkbook, and placed the checkbook back inside. I put her purse down so I could hand her a pen and held the check steady for her to scribble her signature. While she did that, Butter placed the purse back on the chair. That task completed, Butter returned to Ellen and again lay across her legs, as happy as could be.

I watched all of this with awe. "Does he cook and clean, too?" I asked.

Ellen laughed and told me that he responded to over one hundred commands, from answering the door to turning off the lights to sounding an emergency alarm.

He had a job to do, and he did it with the utmost professionalism.

Theirs was a bond that was almost incomprehensible to any observer because it existed on so many intimate levels. Sweet Butter was Ellen's everyday companion, her caregiver, her emotional right hand, her assistant, a close and constant witness to the relentless progression of her disease, her solace, her soul. And she, in turn, was his purpose.

As humans, we talk a lot about the importance of having a life purpose, and ask, "What's my *why?*" Science shows that the emotional benefits of knowing your purpose are magnified if it serves others. Butter's noble purpose—caring for Ellen—clearly benefited him. But he wasn't just a working dog, for an essential aspect of his work was to love and to be loved by Ellen. And anyone who spent time with this pair could see how happy that made him.

Michele Kleier, a real estate broker who was an old friend and client, was calling me hourly for the lab results for Lily, one of her three Maltese dogs, even though I had promised to call her as soon as they were back. Lily's urinary tract symptoms had not improved with the antibiotics I'd prescribed, and I feared that her problem was something more serious than an infection.

As soon as the results were in, I phoned her back. "There are high numbers of both red and white blood cells in her urine but no bacteria, so she doesn't have an infection. I am concerned about some abnormal cells, which are suggestive of bladder cancer. I'm scheduling an abdominal ultrasound."

The ultrasound results showed Lily's bladder wall was both thickened and irregular. Her problem was likely a bladder cancer called transitional cell carcinoma. Lily would need surgery to confirm the diagnosis and remove as much of the cancer as possible, probably followed by six months of chemotherapy.

Back at Park East, whenever any of Michele's dogs were hospitalized, she slept overnight on the waiting room couch using her Chanel purse as a pillow and her coat as a blanket because she thought her dog would be comforted by her presence. So when Lily's surgery was scheduled, I arranged for Michele to bed down in the hospital waiting room overnight as usual.

Lily went through the surgery like a champ. She tolerated her chemo treatments without incident, barking with frenzy along with her sister Daisy each time I arrived to give her the IV, and she went into remission.

But her cancer story didn't end there. She had two more incidents: a plasmacytoma in her mouth and a recurrence of bladder cancer. I didn't even try to persuade Michele to sleep at home for either surgery. The hospital staff simply set up her sleeping area. They did the same thing when Lily needed a benign liver mass removed a couple years later.

This amazing little Maltese survived four surgeries in just three years. And throughout it all, her spirits never flagged. Maybe for another dog or for another family, it would have been right to put Lily to sleep. But not for this dog and not for this family. Neither complained, and Lily never objected to her tests or her treatments. They were devoted to each other, and neither wanted to call "time."

Inevitably, Lily the Wonder Dog's time did eventually run out. At fifteen, she went into heart failure. The dog with nine lives might have died from her first bladder cancer or from any of the subsequent cancers or surgeries, but thanks to medical intervention and her intense bond with Michele—not to mention Lily's own fortitude—this family got five extra years of love together. Michele would have had me move heaven and earth for just another day, and I would have been glad to try as long as that little white tail wagged when somebody looked at her or said *"Lily!"* in her direction.

I have seen the bond between people and pets help to stave off the ravages of illness and prolong life on both sides of the relationship. Sometimes, what happens seems like divine intervention, it is so hard to believe.

Not too long after meeting Butter, the service dog, I was contacted by an animal shelter in Upper Manhattan. They had an adult female black pug who had been found the night before dangerously wandering in traffic on the George Washington Bridge. They were at capacity and couldn't take her. I had a long track record of fixing the medical problems of shelter pugs and, once they were healthy, finding forever homes for them. I agreed to take her on.

All my rescue pugs get names that describe their unique situation, and I named this little girl "Bridgit." Miraculously, her medical issues were minor, and her temperament was unbelievably sweet. I couldn't understand how she could have been abandoned like that. Once she was spayed and vaccinated, I turned to the long list of people looking to adopt a pug.

I called Eric, a thirty-two-year-old man who lived in upstate New York.

Eric explained, "I'm looking for a dog to be a companion for my two little girls. My wife, Stacy, recently had cancer surgery, and she's not doing well. My girls are so depressed, and I thought a pet might bring some happiness into their lives." He continued, "I had a pug when I was little, and he brought extraordinary happiness into my life when I was troubled. I'm hoping this little pug could help us."

I knew Eric was the right person for Bridgit, and Bridgit was the right dog for the little girls. I arranged the adoption, and he drove the two hours into the City to pick her up. When I handed her to him, I was delighted to watch her immediately curl into his arms. I couldn't wait to hear what happened when he brought her home to his two little girls, ages six and eight.

A few days later, Eric called with an unexpected story to tell me.

"As much as my girls love Bridgit, she didn't really bond with them. On the very first day, she instead went straight to Stacy's side of the bed, where she stays all day. Bridgit even tried to jump onto the bed but couldn't because her pug legs were too short!"

I could tell from his voice that he was smiling as he told me this.

"So, I picked her up and put her on the bed next to my wife. She found a snug spot between Stacy's side and her arm and just stayed nestled in there. Now, she leaves Stacy only to eat and go out. I really think the dog knew who needed her most."

Sadly, I couldn't be their vet because they lived so far away, but I stayed in touch with Eric to hear how things were going.

"She's doing incredibly well!" he happily reported on the phone just a month after the adoption.

"She is a good dog," I said.

"No, I mean *Stacy*! She's out of bed a bit more now and has even been taking care of the kids for the first time in months. And wherever she goes, Bridgit is right next to her."

How did Bridgit know Stacy was the one who needed her? We can only be awed by the power of a dog's intuition. I've seen it enough times both not to be surprised by it and to believe it.

Signs of improvement in Stacy's health didn't surprise me, either. There is a ton of scientific evidence that pets make people healthier. Just by being around pets, humans have lower blood pressure, boosted immunity, reduced stress, improved mood, and eased depression. Eric believed with all his heart that the reason his wife outlived her prognosis by one full year was because of the bond she formed with little Bridgit, a "rescue dog" if ever there was one.

Around the same time, a new client, Benjamin, called the office to schedule a "pre-euthanasia" appointment for his terminally ill Yorkie, Jasmine. It is not uncommon for a new client to request a visit in advance of what will be one of the worst days in their lives to meet me and my team so the person who helps their beloved pet pass is not a stranger. Sometimes it's a long time between our introduction and the final day, and sometimes we decide together that it is best not to wait any longer. I go to these appointments prepared for either eventuality.

It's an emotional toll for everyone at City Pets to be asked to end the life of a pet we don't even know. We've had many discussions about this through the years and the answer is always the same. We do it because it's easier for the families and more peaceful for the patient to be put to sleep at home.

Carida, my vet tech for many years, says each time, "We should do whatever is best for the animal." She cries nearly every time. She's raised her kids on her own by working two full-time jobs with veterinarians, one with me and another at a twenty-four-hour hospital on Long Island. You wouldn't think such a tough, no-nonsense woman could be so sensitive.

Carida was with me the day we met Ben. He answered the door of his two-bedroom apartment in Harlem in hospital scrubs. The apartment was charming: filled with colorful rugs on the floor, vases filled with dried flowers, a bookcase with dozens of framed photos, and the telltale sign of a woman's presence—dozens of throw pillows on a comfy couch. On the walls, there were framed photographs of Ben and his wife. A triptych from their wedding hung over the couch. Pictures of them laughing on a beach, hiking on a trail, holiday dinners with their families, and always their Yorkie, Jasmine. There seemed to be so much love in this apartment, but nonetheless, something was making me sad.

"This is Jasmine," said Ben, as he carried Jasmine from the bedroom to the couch. "She's been really sick for a while. I took her to the vet about a month ago when she first got ill. He did blood work and told me she had kidney failure. I asked about prescriptions, and he said, 'Nothing to prescribe because there's nothing we can do.' I guess I just want to make her as comfortable as possible during her final days. For the past week, she barely wants to eat or to go outside."

Jasmine was lying on her side, and she did look terrible. She probably was terminal. But it irked me that the prior vet didn't give Benjamin any other options last month.

"Are you in the medical field?" I asked, gesturing at the scrubs he was wearing.

"I'm a pharmacist."

Good. He would be comfortable around syringes and administering medication in case treatment was possible. "I'll examine her, and while I do that, can you call the other vet's office and ask them to email Jasmine's last medical record and lab results right away?"

The prior lab results indicated that she was in kidney failure, but she also had an elevated white cell count that suggested she also had an infection.

"Benjamin, your dog is elderly and sick, but from her prior test results I think there might be an opportunity to make her more comfortable and give you a little bit more time with her."

"The vet said she was dying," Ben said, completely confused.

"She is very sick and, yes, she might very well be dying. But I also see things on the blood tests that might improve given treatment. She may not have a lot of time left but it's possible that she could respond and have a better quality of life for a little while longer. If she doesn't respond, we can always come back. But once that's done, of course, you can't change your mind."

I never tell clients what to do. My job is to give them options, present the upsides and downsides—and the costs—and let them decide without judgment from me what is best for them. The options run the gamut from extreme intervention to putting the pet to sleep, with lots of possibilities in between.

The vet Ben originally consulted hadn't given him any options. I think it is wrong to assume what a person may wish to do, about the lengths they might be willing to go to, and the expense they're willing or able to bear to help their pet. My only rule is that the decision must be in the pet's best interest. Ben deserved to know all the options available, and a vet who presumed what his choice would be is depriving him of those other choices.

"I'd like to repeat the blood and urine tests to see how much her disease has progressed," I said. "Then I'll go over with you any treatments I think would help her."

He nodded in agreement. "Do you promise to come back if it doesn't work and put her to sleep? I don't want to prolong her discomfort if there's no way to alleviate it."

I promised I would and then bent down to take Jasmine's blood. Despite his medical knowledge, he turned away as I inserted the needle into her jugular vein and withdrew three milliliters of port wine–colored blood. Carida then gently turned Jasmine over on her back and held her still while I inserted a needle into her urinary bladder. The syringe filled with turbid yellow urine, which I injected into the lab tube. As Jasmine's urine filled the tube, I could smell that the urine had an extremely foul odor. I was sure Jasmine had an infection that was almost certainly exacerbating her kidney disease.

I explained to Ben that because Jasmine was so dehydrated, I would start treating her with subcutaneous fluids right away. Dehydration exacerbates kidney disease.

Because it was cold that day and the fluid bags had been in the trunk of our car, they needed to be warmed to body temperature before giving them. A dog's body temperature is around 100 degrees and an injection of 60-degree fluids would be a true shock to the system. Carida went into the kitchen and made a warm water bath in one of his pots to heat up the fluids.

While Ben and I waited, I tried to make some small talk. I commented on a beautiful porcelain bowl next to the couch that was full of dozens of skeins of brightly colored yarn and knitting needles. "Who's the knitter?" I asked. "I love to knit."

"My wife was the knitter," he said. "It was one of the few things that she could do before she passed."

Was?! Oh my God, why do I always do this? I'm supposed to make clients feel *good*, not bring up personal tragedies. Then again, he seemed like he wanted to talk.

"Jasmine was her dog," said Ben. "They were a pair before I even met her. We never had children, and little Jasmine was like our baby. Jasmine and I were both at my wife's side throughout her illness, and she was on the bed with her when she passed."

Don't cry, Amy. Do. Not. Cry.

This dog, I realized, was not just a dog. She was this gentle man's last living connection to his departed wife. I was determined to keep this dog in better health and alive for as long as I could. I knew I was helping Ben by treating Jasmine.

The fluids were finally at the right temperature, and it was time to start treating Jasmine.

"Ben, I think it's best you watch. If Jasmine is going to continue treatment, you're going to have to do this every day," I explained. Ben looked scared. "It's not hard to do and it's not painful for Jasmine. And by giving these injections, you're making her healthier." Ben's expression changed as he nodded in agreement.

I started the fluid injections, and through the intravenous line I gave her a long-lasting antibiotic as well as an anti-nausea medicine and antacid.

I left pills to stimulate her appetite and told him to buy human baby food, which is both palatable and easy to digest. I gave Ben special syringes without needles and instructed him on how to encourage her to eat by pushing small amounts of food into her mouth. She might be more willing to eat once she tasted the delicious baby food.

I phoned the next morning to give Ben the results of her bloods tests and to check in on Jasmine. He answered excitedly, "I'm not sure if it's my imagination, but Jasmine seems a little bit better."

"That's truly the best news, and I don't think it's your imagination. The fluids and the antibiotics are working. The blood results show a worsening of her kidneys, extreme dehydration, and a likely infection. The combination of treatments she had yesterday are helping."

"I just don't know how I am ever going to give her that injection myself."

"Don't worry. We teach little old ladies to give fluid injections," I said, smiling. "So I know you'll be able to do it."

Carida went back later that day with a supply of electrolyte fluids and needles, and supervised as Ben injected the fluids into the space under the skin behind Jasmine's neck. After a few more of Carida's daily visits, he got the hang of it. Jasmine's urine culture results eventually confirmed that she had a nasty urinary tract infection, which in senior pets, like elderly people, can be a devastating problem. The sensitivity panel of the culture confirmed that I had given her the correct antibiotic, so we had a four-day head start on her treatment.

Ben and I spoke every morning, and during each of those calls, he said, "We're a little bit better. Jasmine is eating the baby food and even wanted to walk outside."

I noticed that he said, "*We're* better." Not "*She's* better."

He described that she was more engaged and now even occasionally played. A week later he excitedly reported, "She's eating dog food on her own and wanted to go for a walk this morning!" After about a month, Ben wasn't calling me as frequently, but I knew Jasmine was doing better since I saw the packages containing another month's fluid supplies prepared for delivery to his address.

For over six months, Ben continued Jasmine's treatment. And during that time, little Jasmine had a good quality of life, and Ben had quality time with her. With minimal discomfort for Jasmine (and Ben), the daily injections extended her life. Working together, Ben and Jasmine had another 180 days of cuddles and conversations, no doubt sharing memories about the third person in their family tryptic whom they both loved and missed so much.

On the day we put Jasmine to sleep, Ben, Carida, and I sobbed together. I knew that Ben was saying goodbye to his wife all over again, by losing Jasmine.

When we lose someone we love, it's terrible to have regrets that you could have done or said more. But Ben did do more and got another six months with Jasmine to fill in those gaps, to do and say everything he needed to while taking the best possible care of her. And he had a chance finally to grieve and perhaps to heal a little more over the loss of his young wife.

By playing a small part in intimate relationships like these—Ellen and Butter; Michele and Lily; Stacy and Bridgit; Ben and Jasmine—I'm privileged to see up close the marvelous, special, wondrous bond between people and pets. It is truly like no other.

Perhaps the greatest bond I've ever had with a dog began when I was in veterinary school. I spent the first two years glued to a classroom chair for eight hours a day, followed by long-night study sessions. Junior and senior years were a bit more fun as they mixed classroom study and clinical rotations, but the days were equally long.

I lived with my cat, Mieskeit, in a high-rise studio apartment in Center City Philadelphia. I dreamed about adopting one of the dogs we spayed or neutered during junior surgical rotation but knew that no matter how much I wanted a dog, I couldn't.

One crisp fall morning during my junior year, already late for my oncology rotation, I was rushing up Spruce Street toward the veterinary hospital. I stopped to catch my breath in the courtyard at the entrance before going in. The courtyard was nothing more than a small patch of grass where hundreds of animals had re-lieved themselves, along with a single, gangly tree. Surrounding the tree was a busy circular drive that had a steady flow of cars, trucks, people, and animals coming and going from the hospital. Just as I was about to go in, I spotted a little pug tied to that tree in the center, alone and shivering. I walked over to pet him and saw a note tacked to the tree above him that read, MY NAME IS OLD MAN. I AM BLIND. PLEASE TAKE GOOD CARE OF ME.

"My goodness," I said as I bent down and petted his head. His demeanor immediately changed upon my touch, his sad, hanging tail springing up into a perfect pug curl. His big brown eyes might not be able to see, but they communicated a clear message: *Please don't leave me here like this.*

I didn't need much persuading. "Old Man, come with me."

It took a few minutes to unknot the leash from the tree, and I walked him into the hospital and tracked down my clinical med-icine professor to look at him.

"He seems in pretty good health despite being totally blind," she said. "I'd estimate he's two years old—not an old man at all." Then she handed me the vaccines he needed so I could administer them. "He's not neutered, so you'll need to take care of that."

I will?

Having missed my first class, I now had a half hour before my next one, and so I brought Old Man to my ophthalmology profes-sor, Dr. Gustavo Aguirre, and asked if he would take a quick look as well. He generously agreed. As he examined Old Man's eyes, he said, "I see this far too often, Amy. This dog probably came from a puppy mill, where they factory-farm dogs. Very little money is spent on medical care, and as a result these puppies have all kinds of infections that could have been prevented if only they were vaccinated." He surmised that Old Man had distemper virus as a puppy. Distemper causes central nervous system disease and is often fatal. If a puppy survives distemper, blindness is a common result.

"It's a shame. He's a cute dog," he said. "Unfortunately, there is nothing to do for his sight at this point."

What am I going to do with him now? At least in the short term I knew what to do. I brought Old Man to the radiology department where there were always empty cages for patients waiting for their X-rays.

I whispered to Jenny, a friendly technician in the department, "This pug is not exactly a hospital patient, but until I figure out what to do with him, can he stay in an X-ray kennel?"

She agreed. "I'll shift his kennel every hour so my supervisor doesn't realize we've got a freeloader."

I rushed to my next class in overdrive, thinking, *I've got to find a shelter that will take him and get him adopted.*

But what if they can't find a home for him?

Will he get put to sleep?

Should I keep him?

Could I keep him?

Of course, I shouldn't and couldn't. I had zero time as it was. I could barely take care of myself, let alone a blind dog. I lived alone in a building that didn't even permit dogs. And I knew Mieskeit would hate him. Nope.

But in the short time I knew Old Man, he'd affected me deeply. It might have been a bit of fuzzy nostalgia for my childhood pug, Duchess, but there was more. This abandoned, scared, blind dog had behaved himself with grace as we poked and prodded, taking his blood and giving him multiple jabs for vaccinations. And every time I touched him, his tail popped up in response into that cheese Danish swirl that only pug tails can do. I made the mental promise that I'd get him into shape and place him with the right family because *of course I couldn't keep him.*

I knew I should have left Old Man in the X-ray kennel that night, but I took him home. I wanted him to have a home-cooked meal and a good night's sleep. As I walked into my building, trying to sneak him past the doorman Armando, he asked, "Amy, is that a dog?"

"He's just visiting," I blurted, and rushed into the open elevator door.

"Riiiight," he responded with a raised eyebrow and a smile that seemed to understand it might be a very long visit.

When Old Man and I reached the sixteenth floor and stepped out of the elevator, I unsnapped his leash from the collar. Following just my scent, he trotted after me toward my studio apartment and stood patiently as I unlocked the door. When it opened, he walked in somewhat jauntily and proceeded to bump his way around every inch of the place.

"Careful!" I yelled too late as he collided with my coffee table. Moving a bit more slowly, he gently bumped into each piece of furniture. Eventually he found the open door to the bathroom, slid across the tile floor, did an about-face, and bumped all the way back to where he'd left me standing in amazement at the entrance of the apartment. Then he sat down at my feet, tilted his head up, and "looked" directly into my eyes for a very long moment. My heart swelled to four times its normal size, and I knew I was in love with this dog.

Old Man must have felt the sudden rush of love, too. He stood, wagged his tail, lifted his hind leg, and urinated all over the front door. *I'm home,* he was saying, loud and clear.

With that display I snapped back to reality. "Don't get too comfortable," I said somewhat sternly. "You're not staying!"

Mieskeit, meanwhile, was hiding under the couch where she had put herself the moment the strange dog walked in. She was entitled to a vote, so at last count, we were two opposed, one in favor, of his staying. "I promise I'll find you a forever home, my little bumper. You deserve it."

Bumper. I laughed. "And now I know what to call you."

Bumper stayed by my side for the rest of the evening, which wasn't all that difficult given the apartment's size. It was remarkable how he knew where I was every minute. His pushed-in nose might have been smaller than other dogs', but it was extremely effective. After just a few hours together, I know he could have picked me out of a crowd.

As bedtime grew closer, I fixed up a cozy nest of pillows and blankets in the kitchen for him to sleep on. Since there was no kitchen door, I set up a barrier of chairs and books to keep him inside because he obviously wasn't housebroken.

It was a restless night. I tossed and turned worrying about my new charge. I finally fell asleep, but something woke me at two a.m. It was a pair of beautiful, unseeing pug eyes staring lovingly at me. Somehow, Bumper had managed to break out of the kitchen barricade, find his way to the bed, jump onto it, and position himself so his head lay on the pillow next to mine.

As we lay there, forehead to forehead, his tiny pink tongue darted out and found my nose. I whispered as he licked, "What am I going to do with you?"

When the two of us awoke in the morning, our fate was sealed. Even though I didn't know how, I would make it happen.

My building didn't allow dogs, and my school didn't let students go to class with pets. I didn't have the time needed to care for a dog, and Bumper, being blind, would need extra attention. And Mieskeit made it clear she didn't want him.

Was Bumper sent to me? He needed me, and immediately I knew that I needed him, too.

At breakfast, Mieskeit became a tad more hospitable and introduced herself to Bumper. *You two are going to be best friends,* I thought hopefully.

In just the few hours he'd been there, Bumper had mapped out the entire apartment layout in his mind and memorized it. He stopped bumping into furniture and clearly knew where everything was. *This dog has The Force!*

In the morning we walked to the hospital for my day of clinical rotations. I observed as Bumper took in the environment in his unique way. He sniffed the air and seemed to be counting his steps, memorizing our route. When we got to the hospital, I brought him back to the radiology department. While I talked to Jenny in X-ray, Bumper did his special bumping survey of the room.

"He just memorized the layout," I explained.

"This dog is a genius!"

"I know."

"He can hang here while you do your rotations," she offered.

I couldn't thank her enough. We hid Bumper like this each day and at the end of the week, she said, "Listen, if you're not sure about keeping him," she said, "*I'll* take him."

"*He's mine!*" I replied emphatically.

But it was more like I was his.

Bumper and I were inseparable from that day on. He was the class mascot. We went everywhere together, including a four-week stay in the dorms in the Pennsylvania countryside where vet students did large-animal training. Bringing a pet was against the rules but we'd been lucky.

When I graduated and moved to Manhattan, Bumper came to

work with me at the AMC every day. And when I worked at Park East, he quickly memorized the walk from my apartment on Second Avenue to the hospital on Park. He'd step down from the curb and back up onto the sidewalk at precisely the right moment as we crossed streets—without any cues from me. My role was simply to say "Careful" when there was an obstacle in his way, and when I did, Bumper would stop on a dime and wait for his next command. Watching him, you'd swear he had normal eyesight.

People adored Bumper because he was a friendly, playful, happy, adorable angel of a dog. And most never knew he was blind.

CHAPTER 5

Animals Bring People Together

 My own love story began because of a dog.

In 1987, after graduating from the University of Pennsylvania, College of Veterinary Medicine (and before working at Park East and then starting my own practice), I was an intern at the Animal Medical Center, a huge animal hospital on the East Side of Manhattan. The AMC is the premier animal hospital in New York and one of the largest teaching hospitals in the country. It looks and functions just like a human hospital—an eight-story building that contains a staff of more than seventy-five veterinarians plus technicians, nurses, administrators, and kennel people. It has different medical departments, such as internal medicine, surgery, radiology, oncology, dermatology, dentistry, and ophthalmology. And it treats exotics: any animal other than a dog or cat, such as bunnies, guinea pigs, mice, rats, boa constrictors, parrots . . . you name it. You never knew what creature or ailment you were going to come across in that waiting room.

On many shifts that year, I was the "walk-in" vet for patients who needed same-day appointments, and those were provided on a first-come, first-serve basis. After I finished a case, I would go to the central landing area, pick up the next walk-in folder, go into the waiting room, and just call out the pet owner's name, always last name first.

One day in February 1988, I picked up a walk-in folder for a puppy who was having difficulty walking, went to the waiting room, and called out, "*Shapiro, Steve.*"

"That's me," said a handsome man, around thirty, with brown hair and blue eyes. I can take in a lot of information at a glance. This guy was well-dressed in a cashmere sports jacket, dark wash jeans, and good shoes. He took pride in his appearance. He made a good living.

No wedding ring!

I ushered him and his Weimaraner puppy into an exam room and quickly looked through the folder with the dog's medical record, which included the handwritten fact sheet Steve had filled out. In the space that asked for his profession, he wrote "real estate."

I asked, "Real estate? Are you a broker? Know of any great apartments near here?"

"I'm a real estate lawyer," he said.

Nice. And from his name, I felt confident that he was also Jewish like me. "Shapiro, Steve" was everything I found attractive in a man. *OK, Amy—back to work.*

"So, what's going on with Valkyrie?" I asked, petting Val's velvet ears.

Valkyrie was a beautiful six-month-old silver-gray female Weimaraner. He said, "When I got home from work today, she was limping slightly."

As we talked, I examined Valkyrie. Some of her joints were

painful and swollen, and she had a fever. I'd been a vet for all of eight months by then and still had a lot to learn. What I did know was that this was unusual and that I needed an orthopedist to weigh in and guide my choice of diagnostic tests.

"Would it be okay if I brought Val to the back for a quick consult?" I asked. "I'll bring her right back."

AMC's chief orthopedist, Dr. Chris Thacher, was former military, very smart and precise, and terrifying to most of us interns because of his sky-high standards. With patients and clients, he had a different demeanor. He examined the puppy and then returned to the exam room with me and Val. With the utmost compassion, he explained to Steve that Valkyrie's limp wasn't from an injury. He suspected an inflammatory disorder, osteochondritis dissecans, which is a very painful joint problem of growing, large-breed puppies.

Val was a model patient when we took blood and did a series of X-rays. "We'll know more when the lab results come in," said Dr. Thacher. "Dr. Attas will call you as soon as we get the results."

Steve brought Valkyrie back the very next morning because her limping had gotten worse overnight. By then, the blood tests were back confirming she had severe inflammation. The orthopedic team took over her case and she was admitted to the hospital for supportive care and additional testing. I would be only peripherally involved going forward and was disappointed that my contact with this Shapiro, Steve would be more limited.

"Can I come visit her after work?" he asked.

"Of course," I said. "Anytime. And if you have any questions, feel free to call me."

The next two nights, Steve came to the hospital and sat with Valkyrie. They weren't pleasurable visits, because, despite the medication, she was still in pain.

Even though I didn't have the time, I sat with him, keeping him company. We chatted easily about nothing in particular. I hoped that talking would help take his thoughts away from his sick puppy. Steve told me Valkyrie was the first dog he'd ever had, other than his beloved childhood dog, also a Weimaraner. He'd had Comet when he was a little boy but sadly his family had to give him away when he was only was five.

The next night, I walked into the visiting room with a large dark purple stain down the front of my white coat. A technician had just spilled a bottle of lab stain all over me and I hadn't had time to change to a clean lab coat.

"Wow, Dr. Attas, your lab coat is vibrant today," said Steve.

"You know, I am sick of wearing lab coats, but today I am glad I did," I answered.

"I'd like to see you without your lab coat sometime. Oh, I mean . . . like outside of the hospital, like over dinner or something."

"Maybe," I said, trying to be coy while my insides were screaming *yes*.

"How do I turn that maybe into a yes?"

"Why don't you call me?"

I couldn't stay because I had a patient waiting. Two minutes later, the hospital operator came on the PA system and said, "Paging Dr. Amy Attas." When I picked up, she said that she had an inside-the-hospital call for me from a name she didn't recognize, a Mr. Steve Shapiro.

I smiled. He'd called from a phone inside the hospital.

I picked up the closest wall phone and was patched through.

"Did you forget something?" I asked.

"As you suggested, I'm calling to see if you would have dinner with me tonight."

I smiled, happy that he'd followed my instructions. "I can't," I said. "I have to work until midnight tonight."

"Then how about tomorrow?"

"I can't tomorrow, either." Hearing his sigh, I added, "I'm not blowing you off. Let's connect next week when my schedule is less brutal."

I came to work the following morning at six and, as always, checked the hospital-wide update sheet—what we called "the clipboard"—to see what had happened while I was gone. Overnight, Valkyrie had died.

My heart sank. Poor Steve. Anytime a six-month-old pet dies, it's tragic. But this was completely unexpected, and I knew from what he had told me, this loss would be especially painful for him. I couldn't fathom so much grief.

I waited until a decent hour and called him. "I'm so sorry to hear about Valkyrie. I just wanted to offer my sincerest condolences."

"I appreciate that. I'm sorry we didn't have a chance to get to know each other better," he said. "This isn't the right time for me. I'm frankly just too sad."

That was the last that I expected to hear from Shapiro, Steve.

Four months later, my schedule was even worse. Now my shift began at midnight, and I worked until the next midday. This schedule was making my already bleak social life nonexistent. On one of those long night shifts, my thoughts turned back to February and the cute lawyer whose puppy had passed away tragically. Breaking one of my mother's courtship mandates—and HIPAA rules had they existed and applied to animals—I decided to call Shapiro, Steve and ask him to dinner.

"Amy! I'm so glad to hear from you!" We talked for a while and, before I could even ask, he said, "Let's go on that long overdue dinner date."

Over our meal, the conversation flowed like the red wine we were drinking—about movies, art, music, and our backgrounds. I told him about my James Herriot–inspired calling to become a vet. Steve told me the story behind his adoption of Valkyrie.

"I told you that I had a Weimaraner when I was really young," he said. "Comet. I loved that dog. When you're an only child, you and your dog are best friends. He was so big that I rode him like a pony. We slept together. We were inseparable. And then we had to give him away."

"I'm so sorry!" I said. "Why did you have to do that?"

He hesitated. "My mom died of cancer when I was five." I must have looked stricken. "It's okay, it was a long time ago. Honestly, I barely remember her illness. What I do remember was the day we moved from Westchester to Manhattan so my father didn't have such a long commute and could spend more time with me, and that was the day I said goodbye to Comet. The new apartment didn't allow pets."

He lost his mother and his best friend Comet at the same time. I wanted to reach across the table and hug him.

Steve continued, "I always told myself, as soon as I graduated law school, got a job and an apartment—you know, became my own person—I would get a dog, a Weimaraner, again. Every year, I'd go and watch the Weimaraners at the Westminster dog show. Year after year, I sat at the ringside, always Mondays at eight a.m., and every year the same breeder won. Last year, I finally got up the courage to approach that breeder, and I got Valkyrie."

Now I understood the true depth of Steve's grief. He wasn't just mourning his puppy, but also his childhood, his mother, and his vision of the future with a dog by his side. I knew that future was still possible. He'd find another dog to love, I was sure of it. "When the right companion arrives in your life, you'll know it," I said.

Our waiter, the last staff member in the restaurant, showed great restraint when he kicked us out at one a.m. Steve walked me all the way up from the Theater District and across town back to my East Side apartment. At my front door, he said, "I had a wonderful time."

"Me, too."

He leaned forward, kissed me on the forehead, and left.

My friends were still on the overnight shift at the animal hospital, so I had people to call at two a.m., all excited about my date. "It was amazing and fabulous, but what does it mean when the guy kisses you on the forehead to say goodnight?" I asked my colleague Brett.

He responded, "Amy, no. Not a good sign."

"When do you think he'll call for a second date?"

"A kiss on the forehead? If he doesn't call in a week, forget about him."

A week passed without a call. I phoned Steve again. He immediately asked me out for dinner on my next available evening the following week. We went to the very Parisian Cafe Luxembourg on West 70th Street and shared white and dark chocolate mousse for dessert. *Trés* romantic. Once again, our waiter kicked us out at one a.m. Unlike last time, I got a real kiss goodnight. On the lips.

I called Brett again and told him, "It was a nice kiss. A warm, nice kiss."

I could picture him rolling his eyes when he replied, "A 'warm kiss'? That's what my grandmother gives me."

Steve and I carried on like this for a while. I'd call him. We'd have a great date, always on a weeknight. And he'd kiss me at my door before leaving. I bit my nails waiting for him to call me . . . but *I* always wound up calling *him*. We continued this pattern even after I left AMC and began working at Park East.

Eventually, he started calling me first, and we went to dinner, theater, and concerts; all the while I was hoping that it would turn into something more. Our relationship deepened. There was more kissing, but he made it clear that we were not exclusive.

But I wanted it to be. It got to the point when I had to say something. "Look, I'm not interested in being one of many. If you believe we have a special connection, we owe it to ourselves to see how it plays out. Otherwise, what's the point?" I asked.

He nodded and said, "Okay. Let's try it."

I took that to mean we'd try being exclusive. At our next date—on a Thursday—Steve and I went to Chez Josephine on West 42nd Street, named after the dancer Josephine Baker, for a late dinner after an Off-Broadway play by the great playwright and first president of free Czechoslovakia, Václav Havel. The restaurant's ambiance was very sexy, with red banquets and crystal chandeliers, like a 1920s speakeasy in Paris. I thought the choice to eat there signified our shift to official boyfriend-girlfriend status.

After entrées and before dessert, Steve mentioned, "I'm going to St. Bart's on business next week, so I won't be able to see you."

On business? Who goes to St. Bart's on business? My stomach bottomed out. "You're going with another woman, aren't you?" I asked.

"No."

"Bullshit!"

He took a deep breath and said, "Okay, yes."

So much for exclusivity. "First of all, I don't get it. I thought we were going to try and make a go of this."

"I've always been truthful that I'm not ready for a serious relationship. When I am ready, I know it's going to be with you. But I'm just not there yet."

Tears flowed from my eyes. Steve kept talking, but I was beyond listening. He was telling me what he thought I wanted to hear, and I didn't believe him. After all, he had just lied to me.

"If you care about me at all, even as a friend, lose my number and never call me again," I said. I put on my coat and went outside. The waitress followed me out to give me a big hug and hailed my taxi. At home, I flopped on my bed and sobbed. I woke up the next morning, still wearing my winter coat, with both Bumper and Mieskeit lying on either side of me.

After the breakup with Steve, I met a Wall Street banker named Larry at a dinner party. We started dating, and the relationship progressed very quickly. Over just a few months, we met each other's friends and parents, and I thought there might be a future. There was one major drawback though: Larry didn't get along with my pets. Every time he slept over at my place, Bumper peed by his side of the bed or on his clothing. Mieskeit hissed when he went near her. These were bad signs. Very bad. But I hoped that it was just an awkward early stage and that, eventually, Bumper and Mieskeit would come around.

For my birthday, Larry made plans to take me to dinner at Daniel, an elegant French restaurant on the Upper East Side. We decided it was easiest to meet at the restaurant since we lived on opposite sides of town. I got dolled up in an essential short black dress and made sure my hair and makeup were perfect.

Just as I was about to leave my apartment, George called from Park East. "Amy, we've got an emergency," he said.

The patient, Jasper, a five-year-old orange male cat, couldn't urinate. Male cats sometimes develop crystals or stones in their bladder. As their urine flows from the bladder through their urinary tract, the tiniest bit of grit can clog their very narrow urethra. Their bladders overfill, and toxins build up in the blood stream. The consequences after twenty-four hours can be dire; a cat's bladder might rupture, and if not, the imbalanced electrolytes might even trigger a heart attack. Besides these potentially fatal events, the cats are in terrible pain.

"I'll be right there."

I was able to reach Larry before leaving. "We're going to have to push dinner back an hour. I've got an emergency."

He said, "No problem. I'll change our reservation. It might save time to meet you at the hospital and we can walk over to the restaurant together."

Within fifteen minutes, I was in the ER at Park East, with Jasper on the table in front of me under heavy sedation. Ideally, I would feel a tiny stone right at the tip of his urethra and be able to massage it loose without much effort. I was not so lucky with Jasper. I had to insert a flexible, hair-width catheter through the tiny opening at the end of his penis, and gently push it forward. I attached a syringe to the end of the catheter to slowly flush in saline in an attempt to dislodge the stone. It was delicate work. I had to be careful not to put more pressure on the bladder, which was already filled beyond capacity.

At first, I couldn't feel any forward movement with the catheter. And then, suddenly, his urethra unplugged. Slowly, I pulled back on the catheter. As soon as it was removed, Jasper's urine shot out like from a fire hose due to the pressure of his too-full bladder. It soaked my hair and face, saturated my lab coat and the black crepe dress underneath. This urine had been festering in a cat's bladder for over a day. It did not smell like the Chanel No. 5 I was already wearing.

Clearly, I couldn't go to the restaurant like this. I had to go home, take everything off, put my clothes in a plastic garbage bag bound for the dry cleaners, take a scalding hot shower, and wash my hair three times.

I walked out to the waiting room to find Larry sitting on the comfy couch. He got a whiff and one look at me, reared back, and said, "What happened?"

"I'll tell you on the way," I said. "I really need to get home and shower. I don't think we're going out tonight."

The walk from the clinic to my apartment was just a few blocks. I was explaining what had transpired with my patient when we stopped for a red light while standing on the meridian of Park Avenue between the uptown and downtown sides of the wide street. I was just at the suddenly unclogged urethra part of the story when Larry interrupted me.

"You know what, Amy? I can't do this," he said.

"You're right. There's no reason you have to hear about all this. It's gross," I agreed.

"No, I mean *us*. I can't deal with this." He gestured to me with my ruined hair and soiled dress. Before I could respond, Larry hailed a taxi, got in, and sped away. Just gone.

Jasper went on to make a full recovery, but my relationship died right there. I never did get the Peugeot bicycle that had been sitting gift-wrapped in Larry's apartment for the last two weeks. Dumped, in the middle of Park Avenue, at night. I should have known it wouldn't last. Bumper never liked him, Mieskeit never liked him. My pets were excellent judges of character.

For a while after this I just focused on work, and nothing but work. In early July, I went to the now-defunct Henri Bendel's department store to buy a birthday gift for a friend. I could have gone to Bloomingdale's or Macy's but instead I went to Bendel's. The store happened to be located across the street from Steve Shapiro's apartment building. I bought my friend's present and, on my way back to work, it was as if my feet had a mind of their own, and they walked me right into his lobby. It had been months since our breakup at Josephine's. *It would be nice to see him*, I thought.

And then I regrew a backbone and ran out of the building. Unseen, I hoped. *What was I thinking?*

Within fifteen minutes of returning to Park East, Yvonne, Park East's receptionist, buzzed me. "Dr. Amy, I have Steve Shapiro on the line for you," she said.

I gave in and picked up. "You saw me."

"Saw you? What are you talking about?"

"You didn't see me?"

"I'm confused," he said. "I'm in Maine. I've got airplane tickets with your name on them. I hope you'll fly up for July Fourth weekend."

He's asking me to go away for the weekend after months of silence? How about a coffee first? But was it karma he called me right after I went to his building?

"I'm going to Fire Island with friends," I replied.

"In case you change your mind, I'll messenger the plane tickets to your office," he said.

I asked friends what I should do, and the general feeling was that if I went up to Maine, I'd be giving that guy a "get out of jail free" card, and I'd be nuts to do that.

I went to Maine. The first two days of the weekend were fabulous. We took long bike rides, hiked to a historic lighthouse, ate lobster rolls and blueberry ice cream. I felt myself falling for Shapiro, Steve all over again. But on the third day, St. Bart's came up—it might have been me who brought it up—and I got upset about it all over again. It wasn't pretty, and now I couldn't stay for the last day of the long weekend. I packed my bags and taxied to the airport.

Back in the City, unpacking my stuff, I realized I'd left my makeup bag under the bathroom sink in Maine. *Damn.* On my $40,000 salary, I couldn't afford to replace all the items I'd been collecting over the years. I swore I'd never call Steve again, but I needed my stuff back.

I dialed the rental house in Maine and said frostily when he answered, "I left my makeup bag under the bathroom sink. Can you please bring it when you come? Just leave it with your doorman, and I'll pick it up."

He replied, "I'll give you back your makeup bag, but only if you go to the opera with me. And have dinner with me before the curtain."

It was outright emotional blackmail, but I agreed to the plan. Try as I might, even though I was furious with him and felt like a sucker, I'd fallen in love with him. I kept picturing his face when he learned his puppy was far sicker than he thought. He'd been devastated. He'd loved his dog with his full heart, and if he let himself, maybe he'd love me that way, too.

But this was it. One . . . last . . . chance.

We went to Café des Artistes, perhaps the most romantic restaurant in the City right near the Metropolitan Opera House, its walls covered with lush murals of nudes frolicking in the forest and with low-lit corners for intimate dining. We shared their mouthwatering dish, Salmon Four Ways, and a delicious white wine. Lulled by the food, the lighting, and a contrite Steve, I forgave him for every real and imagined hurt.

The opera—for the life of me, I can't remember what we saw—went by in a blur. Steve spent the night at my apartment for the first time. In the morning, when we woke up, Bumper hadn't peed on Steve's clothes but instead was snoring—on the bed—wedged between us, and Mieskeit was purring away sleeping on Steve's head. Theirs were the votes of confidence I needed.

From that night on, Steve and I have never been apart. We got engaged soon after and married several years later. He fell as deeply in love with my pets as he had been with his. We sleep holding hands decades later. Animals brought us together and cemented our connection for many good years—and many pets—yet to come.

Many of my friendships with clients are based on our mutual love for animals. (I'm suspect of people who openly admit they don't like dogs or cats.) And sometimes, those relationships bring people together in surprising ways.

Back in the 1990s, Al Goldstein, the scruffy publisher of adult entertainment tabloids *Screw*, *Smut,* and *National Screw*, was a New York City icon. Since the mid-1970s, he'd hosted a notorious and boundary-breaking public access TV show on Channel J called *Midnight Blue*, a daring showcase for porn stars, dominatrices, call girls, escorts, D-list celebrities, and a ragtag assortment of fringe New Yorkers. A regular segment on *Midnight Blue* was called "F*ck You," which Al devoted to hotly roasting whomever he was angry with that week.

Al had a pet Vietnamese potbellied pig named Porky—he was

early in that particular pet trend—that he brought to Park East for care. At the hospital, we rarely saw patients that weren't dogs and cats, but Al and his wife, Patty, also had a Yorkie named Heidi, so Dr. B. agreed the hospital would care for their pig, too.

Dr. B. jumped at every opportunity to talk to the press about his being a Vet to the Stars. He gave interviews about working with his famous clients, and one time said something like, "I treat Al Goldstein's pig, and it makes sense he has a pig because Goldstein himself is a pig."

I was shocked he'd said that. Al was in fact a very nice man. In all my dealings with Al and Patty, they couldn't have been more respectful and kinder to me or loving to their pets. And what could possibly be the logic of insulting a client, much less in the press, especially one with his own TV show and a platform for fighting back?

Indeed, on the next *Midnight Blue* "F*ck You" segment, Al *held up a photo* of Dr. B. and said something like, "I want to talk about this motherf*cking a**hole, Dr. B. He owns the Park East Animal Hospital. I took my pets there, and this guy was a total piece of s**t to me." Then he put a photo of Dr. B. on his desk and right on air plopped an actual piece of dog poop directly on Dr. B.'s face. He finished off the segment saying, "Oh, and there was a cute vet there who was great. Dr. Amy. If you go to this hospital, see Dr. Amy."

Al actually did *two* segments about Dr. B. and mentioned my name in both. I'd never seen *Midnight Blue*, but many of my clients were big fans, and they all told me about it, and I got lots of new clients as a result of the hoopla. They all said Al sent them.

In the immediate aftermath of that first "F*ck You" segment about Dr. B., Al seemed to want to befriend me outside the hospital setting. He invited me and Steve to the informal salon brunch that he hosted every Sunday at a restaurant on Third Avenue not far from his townhouse. The first time he invited me, I was in Florida visiting my parents. The next time, I was working. If I didn't accept an invitation soon, he might be offended. I was afraid I'd wind up on his hit list and be featured in a "F*ck You" segment of my own, as I heard that he had done just that to someone else who never accepted his invitations.

So the third time he asked me to the brunch, we went. I was a young, innocent, perpetual good girl who'd never seen an X-rated movie much less been exposed to the City's demimonde. Seated on my right at the brunch was a tall dominatrix in a black patent-leather bustier, thigh-high boots, draped chains, and a sweeping purple ponytail. To my left was Grandpa Munster, the actor Al Lewis who played the role on *The Munsters*. Across the table sat a bevy of beautiful porn stars and probably all the silicon in Manhattan.

The guests were not my own usual Sunday-morning crowd, but brunch is brunch. From the penthouses on Park Avenue to the seedy underbelly of New York, everyone loves mimosas and eggs Benedict. We sat and ate and had a very lovely time.

About halfway through the meal, a late arriver showed up. He was short, hirsute, and unattractive, with an unkempt mustache and a scraggly mullet. As soon as I saw him, I thought, *This guy looks oddly familiar.*

Al Goldstein got up to welcome him, and walked the man around the table so he could introduce himself to everyone. When he got to us, Al said, "Steve, of course you know Ron Jeremy."

Steve stood up to shake Ron's hand and said, "No, I don't think I do."

I heard a few disbelieving snickers from around the table and had no idea what they were laughing about. Al looked at Steve and asked, "Are you pulling my leg? *You don't know* Ron Jeremy?"

"Nope, sorry."

Al turned to me and said, "Amy, this is Ron Jeremy. I'm sure *you* don't know him."

I said, "Hi, Ron. You do look familiar. Don't I know you from somewhere?"

Now everyone around the table was cracking up. Steve, no? Amy, yes?

Al said emphatically, "Come on, Amy, you don't know Ron!"

"Your face is so familiar to me," I insisted. "I'm sure I know you."

Grandpa Munster choked on his home fries from laughing. Even the dominatrix cracked a smile.

Finally, it hit me. "Did you go to Benjamin Cardozo High School?" I asked.

Ron broke out in a grin. "Are you from Bayside?!"

Turns out, we went to the same high school, and Ron Jeremy was the best friend of my next-door neighbor. The mystery solved, Ron and I grinned over the small-world coincidence. My table-mates were still laughing, but I had no idea why. When we got home after the brunch, we did a little research, learned of Ron's legendary physical stamina in the porn industry, and were now in on the joke.

I looked forward to time with Al and visits to his townhouse. Some people might look at Al Goldstein's appearance, his colorful language, the content of his publications and media, and make disparaging assumptions about him. They would be wrong. Al was brilliant and so very important in pushing First Amendment rights. Many important First Amendment cases were in fact generated by pornographers. Al was also a student of history and a total news junkie. We had many fantastic intellectual discussions that helped me see the world in a new way.

In the best of all possible scenarios, animals bring people together to right wrongs. By making a key connection through a pet, I was able to do just that.

It all started in the early 2000s when the head concierge at the Ritz-Carlton hotel on Central Park South called City Pets. The Ritz is a very pet-friendly hotel, and the concierge had sent a few cases to me before. Occasionally a guest's pet would get sick while staying there, or guests were in New York en route to another destination and needed an accredited veterinarian to sign travel papers. Either way, in-hotel veterinary exams were very convenient for the travelers.

I was doing administrative work in the office when the call came in. Carida passed the phone to me and said, "You should probably take this call. It's about a VIP."

Sure enough, the concierge said, "One of our guest's dogs is limping, and he would like to have the animal examined in his hotel suite. I would really appreciate it if you would do it today. This is a very special VIP guest."

"Can you tell me more?"

He said, "The patient is a pug."

Now he had my attention.

The Ritz was only two blocks away and this was a VIP (Very Important Pug!). "I'll be there in an hour."

"Wonderful! When you get here, tell the desk you're here to see John Smith."

"Can you tell me who the client is?"

"You'll find out soon enough. He'll be there for the exam. Does it matter if you know beforehand?"

"No. You had me at 'pug,'" I admitted.

I'd gone to many fancy hotel suites to treat celebrities' pets. Sometimes, I didn't even know who they were. Most of the time, the celebrity wasn't there. Elton John had been my client for years, but when I saw his dogs in the living room of his enormous hotel suite, he was always asleep in the bedroom. This time, I was going to meet the mystery VIP right up front.

That day, my associate Dr. Danielle Dalton had the house call suitcase, so Carida and I threw together some spare equipment to make an exam pack, along with the likely meds needed for a limping dog. We headed to the Ritz.

We walked to the front desk, mentioned John Smith, and were escorted to a small elevator that took us directly to the penthouse suite. I rang the doorbell. While we waited for the mysterious VIP to answer, Carida and I smiled at each other with anticipation. *Who was it going to be? What if we don't recognize him?*

The door opened, and the client was standing there with a cell phone to his ear. He said into it, "Hold on." Then he held out his hand to greet us. "Hi, I'm Bill. Thanks for coming so quickly."

"Nice to meet you, *Bill*," I said. Inside, my thoughts were screaming, *Holy moly! It's Billy Joel! BILL-Y JOEL!! Looking and sounding exactly like . . . Billy Joel!!!*

I am a huge, longtime, genuine Billy Joel fan. My brother Lew had a driver's license when Billy Joel was first becoming known, and he would drive me and our friends to all the small venues that Billy performed in, like the Bottom Line, a tiny club in the Village. When Billy started playing arenas and stadiums, I went to every concert I could.

He motioned us in and directed me to a large round table where we could set up our exam equipment. The suite was enormous, and my working area in the corner had sweeping views of Central Park. There was even a grand piano in the living room. I was introduced to his companion, Katie Lee, a pretty brunette, sitting on the couch.

Billy finished his call and came over. "She was fine this morning and when we came home from our walk, she couldn't put her back right foot down."

He was referring to Fionulla, an adorable black pug, who was three-legged with her right rear leg held up at a 45-degree angle. It didn't seem to slow her down as she ran around the suite with her curly tail wagging.

I picked her up and placed her on the dining table. As I began the physical of this beautiful dog, I stealthily examined Billy, too. He wore dark jeans with a belt, a shirt and sweater both tucked in, and was immaculately groomed. His mustache-goatee combo was so perfectly done, I thought he must have gone to a barber that morning—or rather, had the barber come to him. Not too tall, he was broad and muscular, a solid wall of a person. I found myself staring at his prized fingers that made such amazing music on the piano.

Since I had never met Fionulla before, I did a complete exam rather than just starting on her lame leg. I reached into my bag for my stethoscope and realized with total mortification that in our haste, we forgot to pack one. I caught Carida's eye and silently mouthed, "No stethoscope."

She gave me a look that said, "I got it." Reaching into the bag, she took out the blood pressure monitor headphones, a Y-shaped contraption that looked sort of like a stethoscope. The tube would normally be plugged into the machine, but I placed it against

Fionulla's chest and put the other ends in my ears as if I were actually listening to the dog's heart while instead my own heart pounded in terror in fear of being found out for the ruse.

Yes, I totally faked it.

I finished the exam, and asked, "How long are you going to be in New York?"

"A couple of days," he replied.

Good.

"Fionulla has a patella luxation. The patella is her kneecap," I explained. "The kneecap normally rides up and down in a groove on the leg as you extend and flex it. Same as in people. Fionulla's kneecap is popping out of position, and when it does, she needs to hold her leg up to feel better. You know the creepy feeling when your kneecap pops out a little bit when you are going up the stairs? That's what Fionulla has. It's common in small-breed dogs. I've put it back in the correct position but if the ligaments are stretched, it may not stay, and if it is a chronic problem, there is a surgery to fix it."

"Is she in a lot of pain?" he asked.

"Right now, it doesn't hurt at all." In fact, she was walking on all four feet properly.

I described to him the treatment plan that included an anti-inflammatory injection, oral anti-inflammatory pain medication, and rest. "I'd like to come back tomorrow to make sure that her kneecap has stayed in its normal position," I said. The kneecap was going to be fine, but I could not give this dog a clean bill of health without also listening to her heart and lungs with an actual stethoscope. "No extra charge," I added guiltily.

Carida and I returned as promised. With relief, I found the dog's heart and lungs to be completely normal, and her patella was still in place.

I went home the first day with a story to tell Steve and Marta, our assistant. But before I could get my story out, Marta went first, saying, "You will never guess who I ran into today! I was walking the dogs on Central Park South, and a man with sunglasses and a baseball hat ran over to pet them. He told me he had pugs, too."

"Was it Billy Joel?" I asked.

"How did you know?"

The same day I met Billy Joel's dog, Billy Joel met my dogs. Now that's Manhattan karma.

From that day on, whenever Billy was in the City, he called me to examine his dogs. If one of them was sick when he wasn't in town, he arranged to have them sent in, whether by limo or helicopter, from his home in Long Island. Over time, Katie, the pretty brunette, became his fiancée and eventually his wife and a friend of mine.

Katie called me out of the blue one day to ask me a favor. "Do you know how I could get tickets to go to the Westminster dog show? I've never been, and I've always wanted to go."

"Of course I know how to get tickets," I said. "Better yet, why don't you come with me? I'm one of the official veterinarians for the dog show!"

Katie met me at the employee entrance at Madison Square Garden, and I brought her backstage and gave her an all-access tour of the proceedings. "I've been in this very arena at least five times to see Billy in concert," I said.

"I haven't yet heard him perform in a major arena," she said shyly. I was surprised. I took her to the wall backstage where they have photos of the famous people who played here. It was dominated by photos of Billy. We had a fun day together, and it changed our relationship from client-and-vet to a friendship lasting to this day.

Then and now, I work with the Wildlife Conservation Society (WCS) as a fundraiser for its Wildlife Health Program, connecting their skilled conservationists from all over the world with New Yorkers who love animals and have the wherewithal to make a difference by funding their projects. For one event, I convinced the WCS to lend me the Central Park Zoo and front some money so I could host a party where WCS's wildlife veterinarians would meet some of my interested clients. These vets were doing just what I do—treating sick animals in their homes—except their patients were wild and their homes were on the Serengeti or in Patagonia, not on Park Avenue. The event was a huge success. It raised hundreds of thousands of dollars for the Wildlife Health Program and made WCS lots of new friends that continue to support the organization decades later.

I've also organized themed evenings to educate my clients about WCS's conservation efforts for signature species such as tigers and elephants. At one, I invited Katie to a dinner focused on elephants because I knew from photos in her home that she was particularly fond of them. She, along with one hundred other guests, came for the event at the Core Club, a private club in Midtown Manhattan.

The presentation included WCS elephant experts explaining the dire situation elephants are in due to land use changes and the ongoing slaughter of elephants for their ivory tusks. Approximately *ninety-six elephants are murdered each day* because of ancient and incorrect claims of tusks' medicinal value as well as for their carved beauty. Losing ninety-six elephants each day—*over 35,000 elephants per year*—is simply not sustainable for this critical species. Elephants will become extinct without radical intervention.

After the talk, I arranged for a dozen special guests to stay for dinner in a private room for further discussion with the WCS scientists and conservationists. I sat Katie next to John Calvelli, WCS's executive vice president of public affairs. Although he hoped that she'd make a generous contribution, I was hoping that she could do more. Billy Joel was friendly with Andrew Cuomo, then governor of New York State. New York was at the time the second largest world-wide seller of ivory, and Governor Cuomo could help put a stop to that by signing stalled legislation banning such sales. If Katie talked to Billy and Billy talked to Cuomo, maybe we could do something about New York's ivory trade once and for all.

At the end of the evening, Katie thanked me and said, "I learned so much. I'm devastated about what's happening to elephants. How can I help?"

"There's a lot that you can do," I said. "You have connections that can really make an impact."

Katie jumped on it and was able to put the wheels in motion that led to a meeting between leaders of WCS and Governor Cuomo and his advisers, including the commissioner of New York's Department of Environmental Conservation. WCS explained the need for an outright ban on ivory sales in New York State. I heard that Cuomo asked the DEC commissioner, "Can I do that? Should I do that?"

Indeed, he could and should, and he did. Cuomo signed the bill into law, making it illegal in New York to sell ivory from elephant tusks or rhinoceros horn with rare exception. And Billy Joel did his part to reinforce the ivory ban by putting out a public statement that read:

> I am a piano player. And I realize that ivory piano keys are preferred by some pianists. But a preference for

ivory keys does not justify the slaughter of 96 elephants every day. There are other materials which can be substituted for piano keys. But magnificent creatures like these can never be replaced. Music must never be used as an excuse to destroy an endangered species. Music should be a celebration of life—not an instrument of death.

He also filmed a public service announcement to support the campaign called "96 Elephants." I was so proud of him.

I took great pride in my part to make this happen. Here, love of animals brought the right people together for the finest of reasons.

Years went by. Katie Lee and Billy eventually divorced, and I continued to treat both of their pets, even though Billy was spending more time in Florida. Once, when Steve and I were in Florida to visit my parents, Billy invited us to spend an afternoon at his new mansion on the Intracoastal Waterway just south of Palm Beach.

Somehow, we fell into a conversation about elephants. Billy said, "I don't know if you know this, Amy, but I'm really involved in elephant conservation. I made a PSA for the Wildlife Conservation Society about banning ivory sales."

I smiled. "Did you really?" I asked. "I'm sure that had a great effect."

I'm pretty sure he didn't know about my role in getting the ivory-ban legislation signed, much less that I'd orchestrated his involvement. I never told him. Until now.

CHAPTER 6

There's No Such Thing as a Disabled Pet

I think humans fear disabilities because they worry about how it will limit them, socially, physically, and emotionally. But animals don't care about how they look or what's wrong with them. They don't even know. They simply live their lives to the best of their abilities. Bumper was a perfect example of this.

While I was working at Park East, my patient Dolly Smith, an eight-year-old cocker spaniel, came in constantly with never-ending, painful, smelly ear infections. Cocker spaniels and other dogs with long, furry ears are prone to nasty ear infections because their floppy ears cut down air flow in the canal. Bacteria and yeast—picked up from swimming, scratching, rolling in the dirt, and just normal living—colonize inside the ear in a warm, moist environment, a great recipe for an ear infection. In Dolly's case, her infections were chronic, painful, and frequent.

"It's back. And this time, it smells like *really* sour milk," Mrs. Smith told me.

The smell is so specific that I can detect a bad ear infection by smell as soon as I enter a room.

Dolly was still on the antibiotics I gave her based on the results of her last culture, but obviously they were no longer working.

"I'm at my wit's end. I don't think she will ever get better," said Mrs. Smith. "Now she won't even let me put the drops in. And worse, I think she's going to bite me when I touch her ears."

"Let me take a look," I said, gloving up.

"Be careful! She won't like that!" she said, backing away from her own dog.

Gently, I turned Dolly's left ear back and looked in the ear, which was now a raging infection site. The cartilage folds that should be pink, smooth, and dry were red, swollen, and oozing pus. The swelling was so severe that I couldn't position the otoscope into her ear canal to see any deeper. And her other ear was almost as bad. With this level of inflammation and swelling and the irregular mushroom-like growths that had developed, not only was she in excruciating pain, Dolly could no longer hear.

Mrs. Smith had not neglected her cocker spaniel. She'd followed all my advice to keep Dolly's ears clean and dry, to shave fur on the inside of the ear flap, and to lift the ears to encourage air to get in. But with this breed, it is hard to prevent infections, and once they've had ear infections, many dogs are prone to getting them again and again. Worse, each subsequent infection made the tissue even more unhealthy, perpetuating the cycle.

"I shouldn't have let her go swimming at the lake house," she said. "But she just loves it. And I dried her ears with a cotton ball every time, just like you told me to."

"I know. It's not your fault. You can't keep her locked up when it's so much fun to jump in a lake." I paused and went on. "Mrs. Smith, it's time to do the surgery we've talked about." Several times, I'd recommended for Dolly a surgical procedure called a total ear canal ablation where the unhealthy tissues of the outer and inner ear are surgically removed to prevent further ear canal infections.

"Doesn't that mean you're going to cut out her ear canal? Won't that make her deaf?"

"Well, it would make a hearing dog deaf, but Dolly already *is* deaf because of the growths and inflammation," I explained. "When the ear canal is removed, the infection and discharge will go away, and most important, she won't be in pain. You're going to be surprised how well she'll get along, and without pain she will be much happier."

Mrs. Smith started to tear up. "Won't Dolly be depressed? How will she get through life if she can't hear? I know she can't hear now, but after this she will be officially deaf forever." She looked a little confused realizing what she'd just said.

"I know this is difficult, but she'll be a lot happier when she isn't in constant pain. And she'll be able to swim all she wants without ever risking another infection. Her life will be amazing. She will adjust, I promise."

"No. I can't have a deaf dog," she insisted, tears falling.

How could I make her understand that this procedure would *cure* Dolly of the infections that plagued her, take away her suffering, and make her so much happier?

I had an idea. "Excuse me for a moment. Why don't you both have a seat in the waiting area, and we can pick up this conversation in two minutes?"

She walked slowly with Dolly back to the waiting room, and I went to fetch Bumper. He scampered behind me with a curled, wagging tail into the waiting room. Bumper walked right up to Dolly, and they began to sniff each other. Dolly wagged her tail but remained reserved as Bumper pranced around and did a little of what I call a "bug-a-boo" trying to get Dolly to play. It didn't take much time. The two dogs started romping around the room with each other.

One couldn't hear and the other couldn't see.

"What a sweet dog," said Mrs. Smith, a little surprised by Dolly's happy response to Bumper's flirtatious entreaties.

"He is the best," I said. "Quite the lovebug. His name is Bumper, and he's my dog."

"You're so lucky," she replied.

"And," I added, "Bumper is totally blind."

I don't think that registered with her at first, so I let it sink in for a second. Then she looked at me and said incredulously, "Blind? *He's totally blind?* Like he can't see a thing? But he looks so normal playing with Dolly."

"Totally blind," I replied. "And he *is* normal. I've taken some precautions for his safety, but otherwise, taking care of him is as easy as with any other dog. And he's a very, very happy dog as you see. It'll be the same for you and Dolly. The only downside to this procedure is that afterward I won't get to see you both so frequently," I said, smiling. "Dolly will feel so much better, and she won't be averse to your touch because of pain. You will enjoy each other again."

She agreed to the procedure.

The surgery is difficult, and there is a long recovery. Dolly stayed in the hospital for four days, loaded up on narcotics to ease her post-op pain. She went home on oral pain medication, and she did look pathetic in the plastic cone, which prevented her from scratching the surgical site. When I removed the stitches and the collar came off ten days later, Dolly felt a thousand times better than she had in years—and as a result, so did Mrs. Smith.

Losing a sense—however vital we consider it to be—is far from the end of the world for pets. Dogs adapt to their physical changes, and they get joy out of life for years to come despite them. Our human notions about "disability" and "disfigurement" simply don't apply to animals unless we impose them, and those impositions are usually based on our own vanity or on our own fears for ourselves, all of which are irrelevant to our four-legged family members.

Fred was an adorable long-haired miniature dachshund. He lived with Lucy, a single young woman with a famous New York last name, in a fifth-floor apartment on Park Avenue. The building is small by Manhattan standards, only eight or nine stories and with two or three apartments per floor. The twenty or so families who lived there all knew one another, and they were a friendly community.

Lucy had a lot going on. She was finishing college and also had tons of social obligations. I'm not saying she neglected Fred, but sometimes she didn't give him all the time he needed. Often, instead of taking him outside so he could relieve himself, she took him to the building basement to run around and do his business.

She called me frantic one day. "Fred is pooping blood! Really, it's not a little blood. *It's a lot of blood!*"

I rearranged my schedule to head right over. Blood in the stool is a common emergency, but it's not usually life-threatening. This sounded different. Her cry of "a lot of blood" was alarming.

Fred, normally a very happy boy, looked miserable. Lucy handed me the paper towel she'd used to clean up his stool, and it was indeed saturated with pure blood. I checked Fred's mouth and skin and saw that he had significant bruising on his gums as well as red pinpoint spots on his belly that looked like tiny black and blue marks. Fred wasn't pooping blood. Blood was leaking from his capillaries into his GI tract, under his skin, and probably other places.

All these signs indicated one thing, that Fred had eaten deadly rat poison.

"Where has Fred been in the last twelve hours?" I asked. He might have found the poison on a walk in Central Park or on the street.

"That's the thing, he's been here. I've been kind of busy and I haven't taken him out for a walk for several days," Lucy said.

"So where does he go to the bathroom?"

"I take him to the basement."

The basement is a likely place for a dog to find toxic chemicals.

"Fred needs to get to the hospital right away," I told Lucy. "Meet me outside and my driver will take us there." George and I went to the basement to speak with Karl, the building's super. Walking to his office, I passed storage cages where tenants kept their suitcases, old furniture, bicycles, and plastic boxes full of paperwork.

In the corner of the room on the floor, I saw a few green pellets alongside a chewed black plastic box. Karl came to where I was standing, and I asked, "Is this rat poison?"

Karl's face reddened. "I keep the place really clean," he said defensively. "And it's a good building. But I just can't keep the vermin out, even with rat poison. So every month, I use a different brand to vary it up. I put this one down just a few days ago."

"Show me the bag," I said impatiently.

It doesn't matter if you live in a penthouse on Fifth or the projects on Avenue A, every Manhattan building has a rodent problem. Karl went to his office to get the bag of poison. He was still embarrassed when he handed it to me.

There are multiple kinds of rat poison, and each kills with a different mechanism so I had to know what Fred ate to treat him properly. The chemical in this variety was a long-acting anticoagulant called brodifacoum. Ingestion of even a small amount by a dog dramatically alters the process of blood clotting, and eventually they start spontaneously bleeding. It stays in the dog's system for weeks. Fortunately, there is an antidote, Vitamin K-1, but the poison can be lethal despite that. Success depends on early treatment, and I didn't know when Fred had eaten the poison. But his bleeding both internally and externally was evidence that it was already affecting him, and I hoped the treatment wasn't too late.

Lucy and Fred were waiting on the sidewalk when I walked out of the building, but my car and driver were nowhere to be seen.

Where is Frank? Damn it! Why does he do this?

I had recently hired Frank, a retired City policeman, as my driver. He seemed nice enough, and I thought it couldn't hurt to have an ex-cop around. But it only took a few days before Frank got on my nerves. He yammered nonstop in the car about his marital troubles. And every time I got into the car after a house call and was about to use my brand-new tech tool—a cell phone—to return clients' calls, Frank picked up his way-too-personal monologue exactly where he'd left off. I never responded, hoping he would get the message and just stop talking, but every day, between every appointment, while I was trying to talk on the phone or make notes in my records, he blabbed on.

"She doesn't cook. She's always on the phone. *I* have to do the shopping *and* the cleaning . . ." I was surprised he was so helpful at home since he never did anything to help me and George during the day. When I asked for help loading the car, he always declined, explaining it was too difficult for him to get in and out of the car so many times in a day.

But I knew he was perfectly capable of getting in and out of the car when he wanted to. He just needed motivation.

On his second day working for me, I finished a house call and went to the spot where he dropped me off. Frank wasn't there.

Wait, am I in the wrong spot? Just then, he pulled up in front of me and said, "Police were out. I had to go around the block to avoid getting you a ticket."

That was odd. Wasn't there some NYC cop brotherhood about not giving each other tickets? I got into the car and noticed a crumpled Dunkin' Donuts bag on the floor that wasn't there before. Thereafter, several times a day, I noticed new Dunkin' bags and fresh jelly blobs—sometimes purple, sometimes red—staining Frank's shirt or still clinging to his chin.

With Fred in dire condition, I was furious that Frank had chosen that moment to satisfy his donut craving. And when he pulled up six minutes later, a new crumpled Dunkin' bag on the floor, it was all I could do not to scream at him in front of my client. George, Lucy, Fred, and I piled in, and we sped to the animal hospital. The whole ride I was seething. For once, Frank read my mood, and he stayed quiet.

Fred's blood tests confirmed a prolonged clotting time, and he was already anemic from blood loss. I started him on the antidote of twice-daily injections of vitamin K-1. He also needed two blood transfusions because his blood count was dangerously low. Fred did stabilize after a full week in the hospital, and he was finally able to go home, but he had to continue vitamin K-1 therapy for two more months before his blood clotted normally.

Everyone in the building was delighted Fred was back home and okay. At the next monthly building management meeting, the residents agreed not to use rat bait in the basement anymore.

They needed a different approach to deal with unwelcome vermin, and I had just the thing. With my help, Lucy's building adopted a tawny, oversized adult tabby named Squeaker. Karl and the residents fell in love with him immediately. Squeaker was a natural mouser. It was possible that just his awesome feline presence sent the rodents elsewhere. This solution worked beautifully, and the officers of the building association agreed that Squeaker would be my patient and that they would pay for his care.

I had several other patients in the building, and whenever I saw one of them, I stopped in the basement to say hello to Squeaker. Karl was proud of his new coworker, and he bragged about how Squeaker was keeping the rodent population under control—not to mention what a wonderful companion he was for the staff.

For eight years, Squeaker was healthy and needed nothing but vaccinations. One day, when I came to the building to see a cute orange tabby named Wasabi, Karl stopped me and said, "Something's changed. Squeaker's ravenously hungry even after finishing five cans of food, and still he's losing weight. Early on, I thought I wouldn't feed him a lot, you know, to make him hungry and so a better mouser, but he'd catch a mouse even after he ate everything. Now I'm giving him as much food as he wants but it's never enough."

After Wasabi's exam, George and I went to the basement to look for Squeaker, whom we found napping in the boiler room. I put him on the scale and confirmed he'd lost two pounds despite all that eating. I also noted an abnormal heart rhythm that sounded like horses galloping. I took his blood and the results confirmed my suspicion that Squeaker had an overactive thyroid gland, a condition called hyperthyroidism, which speeds up the metabolic rate; despite eating more, patients lose weight. The increased metabolism also causes the heart to beat in an abnormally fast, irregular rhythm that I had heard on Squeaker. Untreated hyperthyroidism makes patients very sick.

I called Karl and told him Squeaker's diagnosis. "Squeaker will need to be medicated for the rest of his life," I explained. "It's a twice-daily pill and it must be given exactly twelve hours apart. Can you do that?"

He said, "Wow, that's going to be tough. I'll try, but Squeaker isn't always around, and I have so much going on, I can't guarantee I'll be down here every twelve hours. And I don't work seven days a week."

Over the next few days and weeks, several of the building residents agreed to help pill Squeaker, but it still wasn't possible to keep his dosing on a rigid schedule. This presented a dilemma.

"There is an alternative," I told Karl. "Squeaker could go to a specialized veterinary facility and get a single injection of a radioactive iodine, exactly how they treat people with this condition. One long-lasting shot. This treatment would make him temporarily radioactive, so he'd have to be hospitalized for about a week afterward. He can't go home until he's no longer radioactive. The whole thing—the shot and hospitalization—is expensive, around $2,500," I explained.

It wasn't Karl's place to decide whether to take this course because Squeaker belonged to the building association. The residents held an impromptu meeting to discuss the issue, and it warmed my heart that they unanimously agreed to pay the cost of the treatment for a cat that most of them saw only once or twice a year when they got their luggage out of storage.

For the next two years, all of Squeaker's care was routine since his thyroid condition was controlled. But then Karl booked an appointment because Squeaker was limping.

"I thought he might've gotten bitten by something, but he seems to be getting worse. It's been at least two weeks since he put his leg down."

Sometimes, Squeaker made himself scarce for our appointments, which meant a lot of searching behind equipment and in dark basement corners. But not today, and as soon as I saw his leg, I knew he wouldn't be running from me.

"What happened to you?" I asked Squeaker as I gently picked him up and put him on the worktable. His right front leg was indeed not touching down, and there was an angry, hard swelling above his elbow. He hissed when I touched it.

"I can't tell what's going on without an X-ray," I said to Karl. "Can I take him to the hospital?"

"Yes, of course," he said, clearly worried about his colleague of ten years.

The X-ray showed the characteristic sunburst pattern in his bone that meant Squeaker had osteosarcoma, a bad bone tumor. It was a textbook case.

"I am afraid I have bad news," I said to Karl when I returned Squeaker. "The bump is a bone tumor, and it has already caused a lot of painful damage to the bone." I took a breath and continued. "The only treatment at this point is amputation of his leg."

Karl's usual jovial expression deflated. After about thirty seconds of silence, he said, "I can't do that to Squeaker. He's such a proud cat. And how is he going to catch mice on three legs? He'd be a staff member who wouldn't have a job. And the residents won't pay for it, I'm sure." Karl was free-flowing all the reasons why Squeaker couldn't have the surgery.

I said, "Okay, a few things. First, Squeaker's in a lot of pain, and the surgery would end the pain. Second, if you don't do the amputation, the only other option for Squeaker is to put him to sleep because this cancer will spread and cause him even more pain. And third, don't sell Squeaker short. I bet he'll surprise you and be just as good a mouser as ever."

"I have to ask, Doc," said Karl softly. "How much would *this* cost?"

Cost was always a consideration. My job is to be honest, give clients the information, and let them decide how to proceed without judgment. "With presurgical testing, hospitalization, anesthesia, surgery, post-op care, it'll be around $4,000," I estimated the hospital's charges. It was indeed a big number that would be prohibitive for many people, even if the animal in question was an at-home pet. But Squeaker was a basement cat, no one's actual pet.

Karl shook his head and said, "I'll take it to the building board and ask, but I doubt they'll go for it."

"I'm available to answer any questions. And if the decision is to put Squeaker to sleep, I am always here for you," I said.

I spoke to Karl the very next morning. "They went for it!" he said jubilantly. "I met with the board last night and told them everything. The board president said, 'Karl, if this is best for Squeaker, we'll pay for whatever you decide.' As soon as I knew he could have the surgery, I realized I wasn't ready to say goodbye to Squeaker. He's got a lot of great years left in him."

The residents' decision affirmed the basic goodness of people. This sweet cat had served the building for over a decade, and even if, post-op, he couldn't mouse again, he would now get to live out the rest of his life—and maybe even train his successor. Either way, his humans were doing the right thing by him.

Squeaker had the surgery. He healed in the hospital for a few days, and then I returned him to Karl, who continued to care for him in his office. When Karl saw Squeaker on three legs, the big man picked him up, hugged him, and whispered to the cat, "We're in this together."

Two weeks later, I paid them a visit to remove the stitches. "How's it going?"

"He's doing really well! I told Squeaker you were coming and that he should be here to see you, but he ran off. I'll go look for him."

But before Karl could even get out of his chair, three-legged Squeaker sauntered into the office, *jumped* up right onto Karl's lap, and dropped a dead mouse from his mouth *plop* onto the desk, as if to say, "I'm fine; look what I have for you."

"Good boy!" Karl and I said in unison.

A slaughtered mouse is not a pretty sight. But this one was as beautiful as could be.

Squeaker accepted some chin scratches as I removed his stitches. He jumped down with a final glance in my direction and ran off into the basement for more adventures. No one was going to tell this proud warrior cat that a little amputation meant his hunting days were over.

I firmly believe that pets can be just as happy if they are "disabled," and that humans should do their best to help them live their best life. Disabled to us doesn't mean disabled to them, and I've seen some truly remarkable improvements in cats and dogs after traumatic accidents and illnesses. If there is a chance that you can restore your pet to a better quality of life, then why not do it? They'll return the kindness in spades.

When my Bumper was in his teens, he could no longer walk. He had spinal degeneration that made him unable to use his back legs. Steve and I drove to Pennsylvania to fit him for a custom-made walking cart. Bumper was still quite strong in his front end, and with his body resting in the cart and his nonworking hind legs up and out of the way, he could go for long "walks" through Central Park using the wheels as his rear legs. Bumper would wag his tail every time he heard us take the cart out of the closet to put him in it, and he happily used his cart for the rest of his life.

I was grief stricken when Bumper died. He and I had been through so much together. Vet school. My first job. Weekends on Fire Island and in the Berkshires. Boyfriends. Dating my future husband. After Bumper passed, just the sight of his things, including this cart, was just too painful. I put them away deep in a storage closet.

Just a month later, I was asked to be involved in the care of a young rescue pug who was paralyzed in his hind limbs. Here was yet another animal who didn't know that being disabled meant he should be depressed. The shelter was not able to provide the care he needed, and he was transferred to the Center for Veterinary Care for treatment. He would gamely pull himself over to anyone in the room who would give him some love and attention, and, as a result, got abrasions on his belly and legs from dragging his body around. He was going to remain at CVC until he was healthy enough to be adopted. Despite being adorable, young, sweet, smart, and funny, he wasn't going to be an easy dog to place because he would never be able to walk.

I returned home after working with him one day and went straight to the storage closet where I had all of Bumper's things. My eyes welled up, and through the haze of ensuing tears I found Bumper's cart and brought it to CVC the next day.

Providentially, the cart was a perfect fit for this paralyzed pug. From the moment I secured him in the cart, it was as if he could walk again—and knew it. He instinctively pulled it with his front legs and suddenly he was "running" all over the place. Everybody was watching and clapping as he careered about. He even figured out how to navigate hard turns so his wheels didn't get caught, and when he did get stuck on something, he intuitively went into reverse.

I immediately named him Speed Racer, and within days he was adopted by a family who was impressed by his spirit and was taken away to his forever home. I never saw Speed Racer again, but I knew he was happy because it had to be a special family who took him.

We should take a lesson from blind, deaf, and amputee animals to let go of a sense of loss, to live the life we've got, to roll on the grass and savor every treat, with or without slobber. Just like Bumper, Dolly, Squeaker, and Speed Racer.

CHAPTER 7

Daily Life Can Be Surprisingly Dangerous

My dog Cleopatra was not eating. She was one of my rescued pugs, now fourteen and a bit fragile after major spinal cord surgery six months prior. Some days, a little sprinkled Parmigiano Reggiano, fresh roasted turkey, or a slice of cantaloupe would entice her to eat, but nothing was working today. I tried all her favorites and after forty-five minutes, I had to leave for work.

"Steve, can you get your girlfriend to eat?" I called out. "I have to leave or I'm going to be late for my first house call." I often referred to Cleo as Steve's girlfriend because they had a special bond. I wasn't jealous (much).

He came into the kitchen, grabbed an apple, yogurt, cooked chicken breast, and peanut butter from the fridge—some of her favorites—sat down next to Cleo, and said to her, "I'm going to take care of you, my princess."

I kissed them both and left for work.

As soon as I finished my first house call, I called Steve for an update on breakfast. "Any luck?" I asked.

"Yes," he said triumphantly. "I tried everything and finally got her to eat."

I was so relieved. "Great! What did you have to give her?"

"She ate a bunch of grapes."

GRAPES?! Don't panic. Don't yell at him. He didn't know.

"Honey, I'm coming back home. We need to take Cleo to the hospital. I'm sure you forgot—but dogs can't eat grapes," I said very calmly, not wanting to alarm him. I, however, was in a panic.

When I got home, Steve was ghostly white. "I'm . . . I'm sorry," he mumbled, very upset. "I had no idea. I-I mean . . . ," he stammered without taking his eyes off Cleo.

Grapes are poisonous to dogs. In some cases, eating only a few will cause irreparable kidney damage. Other dogs can eat quite a few and nothing happens. The current theory is that the tartaric acid in grapes and raisins is toxic, but the amount varies with the type of grape, its ripeness, and where the grape was grown. Our Cleo already had kidney problems, so eating grapes was particularly dangerous for her.

An elegant lady, Cleopatra didn't appreciate the induced vomiting and three-day hospitalization on intravenous fluids that followed. Thankfully, she made a full recovery. She even ate actual dog food while convalescing in the hospital, but when she came home, she regained her princess status, requiring that Steve sit with her while she ate from a smorgasbord of choices.

Home *is* where the heart is, and your heart might take the shape of a dog or cat. But it is up to humans—pet caregivers, really—to know what is safe and what is not, because our pets are completely dependent on us to do the right thing for them. And often, we don't.

Hazards lurk in the refrigerator, on the coffee table, in the garbage can, the elevator, the medicine cabinet, and even the hanging drapery cords. We try our best to protect them, but it is so easy to slip up and overlook or even create danger for our beloved pets. I've sent many pets to the emergency room because of things their parents did.

They never mean to do it. Their parents all truly loved their animals. But it can be hard to remember that pets, such important family members that we think of them as almost human or even as our children, are still a different species. They do follow different rules. And they are completely dependent upon us for their health and well-being, so having a heightened level of awareness about what affects them must be part of how we love them.

Susan Berkowitz, a medical doctor and author, lived in the West 80s in a brick townhouse with her husband and young children. Her vibe was overworked, frenzied, urban earth mother. A classic West Sider. She was also an adjunct professor at Columbia who'd written a book about the history of childbirth and had four children of her own under the age of five.

A low iron fence with a latch gate in front of their townhouse needed to be opened before knocking on the door. As soon as I walked through the gate, I heard what sounded like a pack of wild dogs barking and growling, but through the thin glass on the front door, I could see just two. The cacophony was created by Chuck, a golden retriever, and Baxter, a German shepherd, both of whom beat Susan to the front door to see who was there.

A few seconds later, Susan, a petite, curly-haired woman carrying a six-month-old in her arms, opened the door yelling, "Quiet!" to the dogs as she waved us into the house. Snarls and growls turned to wags and kisses as we walked through the hallway into the den, which was her kids' playroom.

I scanned for a place to set up, but most of the workable surfaces were strewn with children's toys, empty juice boxes, random shoes, crayons. "Sorry for the mess," she said. "There was no school yesterday. But today, it's just us," she said, smiling at the baby in her arms.

"No problem," I said, reflexively picking up objects like LEGO and small blocks that I thought could choke a dog if swallowed.

Chuck and Baxter were getting each other excited again, each one barking like crazy in response to the other's barking. The ruckus was upsetting the baby, which added to the frenzy. Susan herself added more noise to the room, yelling at the dogs. She pulled up her blouse and nursed the screaming baby, who immediately quieted down. When both the baby and Susan calmed down, it was the signal for the dogs to do the same.

"I'll leave you to it," she said quietly. "The boys are both fine. Just give them a checkup and yell when you are done."

She left, and I started with Baxter, the German shepherd. He was an imposing figure, about eighty pounds of solid muscle, with long gold, brown, and black fur. Some German shepherds are difficult patients, but Baxter was cooperative. He seemed to love my attention, not to mention the cookies after the exams. He remained glued to my side while I did Chuck's exam.

After examining Chuck's eyes, ears, and mouth, I felt under his jaw to check his lymph nodes and was shocked. Ordinarily, the submandibular lymph nodes are small and pliant, just beneath the skin of the neck, but Chuck's were the size of baseballs and just as hard. I checked all the other lymph nodes in his body, by his shoulders, under his armpits, and in his groin. They were all markedly enlarged and hard, though none were visible because of his long golden fur.

I called up the stairs, "Susan, can you come down?"

She was still breastfeeding when she rejoined us in the den. "Done already?" she asked.

"I found something with Chuck."

Her composed facial expression changed, and she removed the almost sleeping baby from her breast and laid her down on the carpet.

"Palpate Chuck's lymph nodes," I said. "Right under the jaw here." I placed her hands in the correct location.

As a trained physician, Susan knew immediately that they weren't normal. "How could I not have felt these?" she asked.

"Goldens have long hair, and unless you happened to touch him in the right spot, you'd never notice."

"What do you think it is?"

"I think Chuck has lymphoma," I said.

Carida was my nurse that day, and like Radar on *M*A*S*H*, she was ahead of me, preparing a syringe for me to aspirate the abnormal nodes. I inserted the thin needle and rapidly pulled back on the plunger of the syringe several times extracting cells, which I sprayed onto a microscope slide. With staining, the pathologist would be able to identify the cells in the sample and confirm my presumptive diagnosis of lymphoma.

Chuck was unfazed, but Susan was reeling from the shock. "If he does have lymphoma," she said, "I'm not going to treat him. I know how sick people get when they're treated for lymphoma. I could never put my dog through that."

"Can we do this one step at a time? Let's get results back first, and then we can decide what to do."

Within twenty-four hours, I had confirmation that Chuck had lymphoma, one of the most common cancers found in dogs. Golden retrievers are one of the breeds most often diagnosed with it. Untreated, it will progress to other organs, such as the liver, spleen, bone marrow, bones, and brain. When treated early, there is a better chance of remission.

In Chuck's case, the abdominal ultrasound and total body imaging that we did two days later didn't detect cancer elsewhere and, given the early diagnosis and the absence of spread, Susan changed her mind and agreed to treatment. I started the chemotherapy.

Chuck was given L-asparaginase, vincristine, Cytoxan, and Adriamycin—the same drugs that are used to treat cancer in humans. Susan knew them from being a practicing physician. She often said how amazing it was that dogs and people not only get the same diseases but were often treated with the same medications.

Chuck did well during the course of treatment. He saw me every three weeks for blood tests and chemotherapy injections, and he was apparently feeling like a normal dog.

Sadly, despite catching his lymphoma early and immediate intervention, Chuck didn't achieve a long remission. I was able to give him only one year of quality life. When he came out of remission and no longer responded to chemotherapy, we agreed to put him to sleep to avoid its worsening.

The whole family missed Chuck terribly, but I know it was Baxter who missed him the most. Chuck had been his best friend and constant companion for years. After Chuck's passing, Susan gave Baxter as much attention as possible to compensate for his loss. She took him for extra-long walks and occasionally let him run off-leash in Central Park to play with other dogs. All that helped. A bit.

One Monday morning, Susan called me in a panic about Baxter. "Dr. Amy, I have no idea what's going on," she said. "Baxter's feet are swollen. He's breathing rapidly and his face seems puffy.

He's lethargic and didn't eat breakfast this morning. And he can't stop drinking water."

"Back up," I said. "Just start at the beginning. How long has he had symptoms?"

"Okay, it started over the weekend. I took him for a long walk in Central Park on Saturday, and then he got into a chase with a Labrador. When we got home, he was limping. I thought he must have strained his ankle or something."

"Is he still limping?"

"No, that stopped after I gave him two Tylenols."

"What?" I blurted. *"Tylenol?"*

"Two on Saturday," she said. "And then he seemed to feel worse, so I gave him another two yesterday."

"What color is his tongue?" I asked.

"Give me a second," she said. There was a pause, and then she said, "Oh my God. It's blue! Is he going to die?"

If a pet has a pimple, the owner always asks that. Ninety-nine times out of a hundred, their alarm is an overreaction to something not very serious. In this case, however, I feared it might not be.

As calmly as I could, I said, "Susan, you have to take Baxter to the ER now." Humans can take as much as 3,000 milligrams of Tylenol a day safely. But *any* amount of Tylenol is deadly dangerous to dogs—and even more so to cats. Along with the symptoms she had described, like facial edema, Tylenol can cause liver and kidney failure as well as red blood cell destruction. It's so toxic, just one pill can kill a cat.

"I had no idea!" she said, her voice sounding increasingly upset. "I saw you use human medicine for Chuck, and I didn't want to get another vet bill, so I just gave him the same medicine that I take for limping."

I can't tell you how many people think they can treat their pet by reaching into their own medicine cabinet and administering a human medicine. I've seen terrible outcomes when clients gave their pets human heart medication, blood pressure drugs, or ibuprofen (which is just as toxic to pets as Tylenol). Because of her own human medical knowledge, Susan thought she could manage Baxter's limp on her own. But an MD is not a VMD, and pets are not small, furry people. A pill that is helpful for a person might end a dog's life.

Since Baxter had been given the pills days before, my options were limited. Induced vomiting wouldn't help because the toxin was now in his system. I couldn't use activated charcoal to absorb it in his stomach because the chemicals were already in his bloodstream. The blood work taken on his hospital admission confirmed he was anemic and had kidney damage, both caused by the Tylenol. He would need hospitalization on intravenous fluids to support his kidneys until they healed and blood transfusions for the anemia.

Baxter spent seven full days in the ICU. The total hospital bill came to over five thousand dollars. "The irony is I gave him the Tylenol because I didn't want to pay for a vet visit," Susan said. I couldn't be angry with her; she was racked with enough guilt about what she'd done. If only she had just called me or even googled "Is Tylenol safe for dogs?" none of this would have happened.

They both survived the ordeal. Susan realized her degree qualified her to treat only certain *bipedal* animals, and she learned a lesson she'd never forget: Just because some drugs work on both people and animals—like the chemo I gave to Chuck—does not mean *all* human meds are safe for animals. She vowed never to treat a four-legged family member again.

My client Charles Hampton, a divorced man in his early fifties, lived in one of Manhattan's finest buildings, on Fifth Avenue in the East 60s. It was designed in 1920 by architect James E. R. Carpenter, and although it had a relatively plain limestone façade, as soon as you walked into the lobby you beheld its splendor. Twenty-foot ceilings, ornate finishes, uniformed doormen, and porters all over rushing to help you with your bags. The building has only eleven floors, each with just a single apartment. The apartments are huge, some with fifteen rooms measuring 7,500 square feet, all of them with glorious Central Park views. One recently went on the market for a jaw dropping $55 million!

Just looking at Mr. Hampton, you would never think that he came from extreme wealth or that his family founded one of New York's largest Wall Street investment banks. He was just a nice guy, a casual dresser with blondish hair and a friendly smile. He was reasonably attractive, but as Joan Rivers used to say, "They're all attractive when they have that much money."

I never saw him at work, where he wielded that wealth and power. I only knew him as the besotted owner of his golden retriever, Lucy.

Every morning from six to seven, Mr. Hampton took Lucy for a walk in Central Park on her flexible leash, locking the extendable leash at a proper six-foot length until they got to the park and then allowing it to extend to its full thirty feet. Lucy knew exactly when he'd unlocked it, and as soon as she heard that click, she ran ahead pulling the leash out as far as it would go and dart back and forth having the time of her life even while still on-leash.

New York law requires that dogs be kept on a leash no longer than six feet at all times. Though the law is clear, there is a long-standing tradition that police rarely issue tickets for long-leash or off-leash dogs in the park before nine a.m.

There is no quick retraction mechanism on a flexible leash, so you must pull back on the leash part in sections to reel a dog back. It's cumbersome and time consuming and is not a quick enough process to pull a dog back from danger twenty or thirty feet away. A dog on a long leash might run ahead into the street and get hit by a car, get tangled up with a bike rider, or mistakenly approach an aggressive dog—all while an owner looks on helplessly. I know of situations where each of these bad things have happened to dogs, and I am simply not a fan of flexible leashes.

One sunny day, as Mr. Hampton and Lucy finished their park play and walked back into their building, the doorman stopped him to ask a quick question. Mr. Hampton unlocked the leash as he always did when they entered the building, and Lucy went off on her usual path to the elevator, which was around the corner of the lobby.

As chance would have it, the elevator door was open and, without anyone being able to see Lucy around the corner, she walked into the elevator as usual. The door closed behind her though she was still attached to the leash Mr. Hampton was holding thirty feet away. The elevator was summoned to pick up a resident from the basement gym, the doors closed, and the cab started downward with Lucy inside still attached to the extended leash in the hand of Mr. Hampton.

When the elevator descended about fourteen feet, Lucy was yanked up to the top of the cab by her collar, still connected to the leash. Only when the handle was forcibly yanked from Mr. Hampton's hand and flew around the corner did he realize something was wrong. He chased it to the elevator door and watched the length of the leash disappear into the elevator shaft and the leash handle itself slam against the closed doors.

The doorman ran to check the elevator security monitor and saw Lucy dangling by her neck at the top of the cab in wide-eyed terror. Thankfully at that moment Lucy's collar snapped, and she fell nine feet to the floor. The doorman summoned the elevator back to the lobby, the doors opened, and Lucy came out apparently unscathed, her tail wagging, looking at her father as if to say, "Boy, that was unpleasant. Let's not do it again!"

Mr. Hampton called me as soon as they got back to his apartment so I could check Lucy. Surprisingly, she had only small abrasions around her neck and was otherwise unharmed. If the collar hadn't snapped, she would have been strangled to death. Although she was miraculously fine, the elevator cab needed new mahogany panels because Lucy's frantic scratching while choking from the ceiling damaged the wood.

In addition to needing a new collar, Lucy needed a new leash. This time, one that was just six feet long.

Some pet dangers lurk quietly in our homes. Even lovely things that dazzle our eyes and please our noses can be deadly to pets. I found this out a few years ago while doing springtime rounds at the Gramercy Park home of my client Violet, a lawyer and mother of two, and her two-year-old cat, Croc. "She's vomited five times this morning," she told me.

I'd examined Croc just a few weeks before and found her in good health, so I wasn't too concerned.

A cat threw up? It must be Tuesday.

A few cat vomiting episodes is not usually something to worry about. Though it is upsetting to see your cat make that telltale heaving posture and the horrible sound of vomiting, it usually is a self-limiting problem.

"It might be a hairball, or maybe she was eating too fast," I said. "I'll come by to check to be sure."

Throughout the day, while tending to my other patients, I was dreading going to Violet's apartment. Croc was a difficult cat. In fact, Croc was short for Crocodile. I couldn't work with her on a kitchen counter or table, as she would coil her body around to try and get her teeth or claws into the flesh of our hands, wrists, and arms, inflicting pain and often drawing blood, just to force us to let her go, and she often succeeded. We worked in the apartment's smallest bathroom so that when we needed to release her, she had no place to hide, and we were able to pick her up again.

Often the most stressful part of a house call with a frightened cat is the chase to get it. Croc was one of the most difficult. On our last visit, my nurse Jeanine, an empathic millennial vegan who was a cat in at least three former lives, and I were locked in the small bathroom with Croc for forty-five minutes—*four* catch-and-releases—just to get a single blood sample. It was a miracle we weren't torn to shreds. I credit Jeanine for that. She has an amazing ability to handle cats, maybe because of her previous lives.

That sunny April day, Jeanine and I arrived with our wheelie full of testing equipment and medication we might need for a routine stomach issue. We didn't bother setting up on the granite kitchen countertop, anticipating another sweaty bathroom wrestling match.

Violet brought her cat over to me, and Croc was uncharacteristically docile. I quickly wrapped her in a towel and took her to the bathroom, thinking, *Good for me—but odd.* I placed her in the sink and started the exam. She was too quiet. Rather than trying to wound us, she submitted to everything we did, including taking blood. She was dehydrated from vomiting, so I gave her fluids and anti-nausea medication. Croc barely flinched. She didn't try to bite me even once. This was not the firebrand I knew. This cat was sick.

After we finished, Jeanine packed up our stuff, and I headed into the living room to speak with Violet and ask my veterinary-detective questions. I was hoping for some clues to understand Croc's symptoms and personality change. Before I got my first words out, I smelled the potential cause, and then I saw it, placed in the center of a glass coffee table in the living room.

"That is a stunning bouquet of lilies," I said, gesturing to the arrangement of some two dozen fresh white trumpet-shaped flowers at full bloom with orange-dusted stamens.

"Thank you," she said. "I got it for an Easter party last weekend."

"These flowers have been here all week?" I asked, already heartbroken.

All lilies, but especially Easter lilies, are deadly for cats. If they take even a tiny bite of any part of the plant—stem, leaves, flower, pollen—virtually irreversible kidney failure results. Many cats who ingest lilies die. Those who survive do so because of quick, intense—and very expensive—medical therapy like in-hospital diuresis, kidney dialysis, or kidney transplants.

I inspected the bouquet, and, sure enough, I saw holes in the petals and leaves that could only have been made by a cat's teeth, as well as a few torn pieces on the coffee table. "Have you seen Croc nibbling at this?"

"She always eats my flowers," said Violet, laughing. "Usually, I spray them with lemon water, but it doesn't always work. Croc is naughty."

"I'm sorry to tell you this, but Croc needs to go to the hospital right away." *If she's been munching on these all week, it was already too late.*

Violet was sufficiently spooked, and on my instruction, she immediately took Croc to a nearby veterinary emergency hospital to begin treatment even before we had blood tests back. A few hours later, the tests confirmed she had been poisoned by eating the lily plant, and, worse, there was now so much kidney damage that drastic treatment would not help.

It's a special kind of heartbreak when a feisty cat like Croc becomes a cooperative patient. It often means that they are desperately unwell. In these situations, I truly long for them to try to bite me again. Most of these snappy cats are sweethearts with the people they love, treasured family members who snuggle, purr, and stretch into hilarious positions. They hate me for a good reason: I stick them with needles. Although I don't like to be thought of that way, I understand.

Croc was a young cat, a beloved family member, and she should have had at least a dozen more years of happy life. But hers was cut short by her owner unknowingly bringing home beautiful—but deadly—flowers to celebrate a holiday.

In some traditions, lilies symbolize life and rebirth, but not in mine. Lilies should come with a skull-and-crossbones warning about how dangerous they are to cats. Many plants are called "poisonous" because when eaten they can make animals sick, which might mean an upset stomach or diarrhea, a far cry from near-certain death that lilies' poison means. No cat deserves to die because they nibbled on Mom's pretty bouquet.

I have been on an anti-lily campaign my entire professional career. If you have a cat and lilies in your home, make a choice and keep only one of them—the cat, of course. And since you are rightfully keeping your cat, get some kitty grass for your cat to nibble and perhaps orchids, which are not toxic, for you to enjoy.

Candy was a three-year-old cat I'd known since she was a kitten. Until this day, she'd never been sick. Her mother, Nancy, called a lot with questions about diet, kitty litter, play practices. She would read cat internet sites and get a lot of strange ideas as a result, and she'd think nothing of calling to ask, "Should I give Candy only bottled water?" or "What's the best kind of hairbrush?" or "How many hours of sleep does she need?" All good questions, I imagine, even if they didn't rise to the level of veterinary care. Nonetheless, while Candy was a pleasure to take care of, Nancy could make me a little crazy.

This time, Nancy called not to ask a hundred questions but to report Candy wasn't feeling well. "She's acting strange," she said. "Several times a day, she goes into a trance. Her eyes get all glassy. She just stares at the wall and meows for a while, and then she takes off running all over the furniture and knocking stuff over, all the while drooling. It's frightening. Do you think she might have rabies?"

"How long do these symptoms last?"

"Like half an hour, and then she's normal again."

These were a weird set of symptoms, for sure, and it wasn't apparent what was going on. But I knew it wasn't rabies. Could this be a central nervous system disorder, a metabolic problem, a parasite, an abscess, a tumor? These would be unusual diagnoses for a young cat, but hers were unusual symptoms.

I went to Nancy's East Village apartment and found her racked with concern. At first glance, Candy looked great. She rubbed against me and purred when I walked in. I did a complete examination with emphasis on her central nervous system, looking for any clues that might help with the diagnosis.

She seems normal, I thought, perplexed. Of course, there were myriad possible diseases that could cause intermittent problems, like epilepsy, and I needed to prioritize my testing. A rare liver disease where the blood vessels are abnormal can cause a cat to have the occasional symptoms Nancy described.

"I'm not finding anything wrong based on her physical exam. I'll take some blood and urine samples to see if there is any indication of a metabolic disease."

"Can I have a few minutes alone with her first?" asked Nancy, wringing her hands with anxiety.

"Of course," I said.

Nancy took Candy into the kitchen. I could hear her crying and telling Candy tearfully, "Don't be sick and *please* don't be dying. I will do anything to make you healthy. *Pleeeaze.* I love you so much."

My nurse Shari and I made eye contact. We didn't need to say a word to send clear messages because we had worked together for many years. An extremely talented technician, I first met her when she was working at the Center for Veterinary Care, before she left to fulfill her lifelong dream of living in Alaska. Ultimately, she moved back east and joined my practice. Our long history gave us an instant shorthand.

Shari was transmitting, *I know this woman is a bit kooky, but I understand that love.* I silently sent back, *Yes, so do I.*

While Shari set up for the blood tests, I gently knocked on the kitchen door and said, "We're ready for her."

I walked in and noticed right away that Candy had a glazed look in her eyes. Then she began to make a funny howling sound and started drooling from one side of her mouth. I reached down to pick her up and right then, Candy went into the hyper phase that Nancy described. She ran out of the kitchen and raced around the apartment jumping all over the furniture. We watched what looked like a cartoon character as she ran back in and jumped onto the kitchen counter, where she crashed straight into a porcelain herb jar that smashed to the floor.

"Quick, grab Candy so she doesn't cut her paws," I yelled. But Candy was already rolling around in the shards and herbs and wouldn't let us touch her. When Candy went into a full, dull stupor, I was able to pick her up and get her away from the broken porcelain.

Nancy was hysterical. "See? I'm not crazy. There's something really wrong."

"You're right," I said. "Let's sweep up the jar and all that oregano before Candy starts up again."

"Oh, that's not oregano," Nancy corrected me. "It's a special organic catnip that I just bought. I read about it on the internet."

Catnip is a plant that is commonly thought of as "pot for kitties." It does have a sedative effect, and in some cats, it can be hallucinogenic. "Candy is on catnip?" I asked. "How long has she been eating this?"

"I got this fresh batch two weeks ago, and she really loves it."

"How often do you give it to her?" I asked.

"Oh, it varies. It depends on how stressed out she is. I mean, just now, to calm her down for her blood tests, I gave her a big pile of it."

Shari stifled a laugh. I just rolled my eyes.

I was glad that I hadn't rushed Candy in for a spinal tap or some other invasive testing. There was no medical problem here. This poor cat was stoned out of her mind, courtesy of her mom and the internet. One of my most difficult diagnostic challenges had just become one of the easiest.

And it did seem apparent that organic *is* better.

CHAPTER 8

Humans Behaving Badly

When I was in fourth grade, I had a beloved fish tank. I decorated the ten-gallon aquarium with a gravel bottom and plastic plants. I wanted to make an attractive and comfortable home for the six zebra fish I'd purchased at the pet store.

The salesman had suggested zebras because they are easy to care for, especially for a beginner fish keeper. He sold me three males and three females, but I couldn't tell them apart. A few weeks later, I noticed that some of the fish's bellies were growing rounder. Eventually they laid eggs in the colored gravel that were fertilized by the males. Fourth-grade-level biology in action! A few days later, innumerable baby zebra fish swam around the tank. And I became a ten-year-old grandmother.

I often stopped at the pet store on my way home from school to admire other species of fish and to purchase supplies. I also needed to buy lots of frozen mosquitoes and larvae to feed my zebras as the babies were now almost adult size. Each time I went to the store, I was drawn to the tank of a real showstopper, a beautiful angelfish. It was the size and shape of a Dorito, with stunning black-and-silver vertical stripes, and I thought it would look great swimming along with my horizontally striped zebra fish. The angelfish was expensive—$2.99—which would blow my entire weekly allowance, but finally I went for it.

The salesman, whom I had never seen before, put the angelfish in a plastic bag, closed it with a pink rubber band, and told me to let the bag float on top of the water for an hour before opening it and allowing the angelfish to enter the tank. I followed his instructions precisely and watched the new fish swim around for a while, then finished my homework, ate dinner with my family, and went to bed.

The next morning, I ran to the tank to see how my new fish was doing. There it was, swimming around. All by itself. Angel was the only fish in the tank! Every one of my zebra fish was gone.

I called out in shock and horror, "Angel ate everybody!"

Those zebra fish had been my friends. For months, I'd taken excellent care of them, measuring their food, scraping algae off the sides of the tank, cleaning the filter, adding just the right amount of chemicals to keep the water clean. And they would have continued living their best fish lives if I hadn't brought home this monster.

Absolutely heartbroken and crying hysterically, I sobbed to Mom, "This is all *my* fault."

She consoled me, but there was only so much she could do. I didn't blame the angelfish for doing what came naturally. But I bought it and put it into the zebras' tank. I believed that I had killed my fish friends. This was a heavy burden for a kid.

I changed Angel's name to Devil, and although I never loved that fish, I took care of it for the rest of its life. I'd signed on to do that when I handed over the three crumpled dollar bills to the salesman. He hadn't asked about my tank and, worse, didn't think to tell me that angels are one of the most predatory tropical fish you can put in a community tank. If he'd given me this warning, I wouldn't have bought it.

The zebra decimation in my fish tank taught me a couple of valuable lessons. Foremost, if you are going to bring animals into your life, you must educate yourself as to how best to care for them. Second, in my career as a veterinarian, I would counsel pet families about what they needed to know to keep their pets healthy. That pet store failed me, but I resolved I would never fail my clients in that way.

This imperative has stayed with me throughout my veterinary career. It is frustrating and even maddening when I advise people about best practices for their pets and they don't listen. An apt equivalency would be if that pet store salesman had told me, "If you put this angelfish in your tank, it'll eat your zebras," and I replied simply, "No, I'm sure it'll be fine."

No, it won't be fine.

You wouldn't think that anyone would *knowingly* put their pet in danger, and yet they often do. Outright disregard by humans for their pets' best interests angers me the most, as it often has disastrous consequences for the animals they'd morally signed on to protect for their entire lives.

Nine months after starting my house call practice, on a beautiful day in May, I was scheduled to visit the Fifth Avenue home of a new client for their two cats' annual checkups. When George and I arrived, the doorman called up to the apartment to announce us.

"Would you like them to take the North or South elevator?" he asked the residents. "And which floor would you like them to come to, the fifteenth, sixteenth, or seventeenth?"

As we rode in the private elevator to the selected seventeenth floor, my head was spinning. A *triplex penthouse* apartment, with each floor spanning the entire building and all with Central Park views? This was truly a palace in the sky. I was still new to house calls, but I already knew that there weren't many homes like this in Manhattan.

The elevator opened into the apartment's grand living room. When I think back on it, the room had the kooky exuberance of the Baz Luhrmann set in the movie *Moulin Rouge*. Colorful and chaotic, the vast space was encased in hunter-green wallpaper with exotic birds and flowers. The room was filled with eye candy: a six-foot-tall sculpture of an elephant draped in an Indian sari; a huge, shiny Jeff Koons teal balloon dog; and an eclectic collection of pricey furniture. There was a Danish modern chaise, a pop-art Lucite coffee table, and a massive rococo red velvet couch with gold tassels on the arms. On the couch sat two large pillows embroidered with the words "The Queen Sits Here" and on the other end "The King Sits Here."

A woman with a blond pixie cut named Betty (the Queen, I assumed) came to greet me with an outstretched, muscular arm. She was petite, very attractive, and impossibly fit.

"*King*, come to the living room. The vets are here," she shouted into another room.

"Coming, Queen!"

Her husband entered, followed by two adorable cats. He introduced himself as Don. He, too, was very attractive and impossibly fit.

They actually called each other King and Queen right in front of us without any sign of embarrassment or irony. I couldn't make eye contact with George for fear I might start giggling.

Their two cats, Roast Beef and Noodles (not Prince and Princess?), rubbed against my pant leg. I bent down to give chin scratches and Roast Beef, a large black-and-white, flopped to his side, exposing his fat belly and purring loudly.

Then another voice called the cats' names from the floor below, and the felines immediately ran down the stairs.

Betty laughed. "Polly is probably feeling lonely downstairs. They always come when Polly calls them." *Who is Polly? Maybe the housekeeper?* Reading the question on my face, she explained, "Polly is our parrot."

Right on cue, Polly, a large rainbow-hued bird, who looked like she came out of the wallpaper, flew into the room and perched on a curtain rod, followed by the trotting cats. Betty coaxed the parrot into its golden cage and then sat down on the couch by the Queen pillow. Don took his spot by the King pillow.

"Have a seat," said Betty, motioning me to the rococo chaise opposite the royal couch. "Let's talk cat." As I sat, my gaze was drawn to the floor-to-ceiling windows and sliding doors that opened onto the wraparound terrace, beautifully planted with flowers and trees.

I began to explain my house call practice and how the exam would proceed. As I talked to King and Queen, I noticed Roast Beef casually walk past us to go through the open sliding glass doors and out onto the terrace. He was followed by Noodles. They immediately began running and playing outside. Before I could get my words out, Roast Beef jumped up on the parapet wall, two hundred feet above the ground, and ran along it.

"Oh my God! *Your cats are on the terrace!*" I yelled, already on my feet, running toward the sliding door.

Queen Betty said, "Relax, they go out there all the time. They love to play outside, so we leave the door open for them."

"No! No, you can't do that. It's incredibly dangerous."

"It's *fine*. We've had cats all our lives. We always let them outside."

I opened my mouth to try again but the look on her face made it clear that the discussion was over.

They might have always kept their terrace doors open and never had a problem before, but that didn't make it safe for their cats. Every year, during the first beautiful days of spring, New Yorkers in high-rise buildings throw open their windows and balcony doors and literally *hundreds* of pets—mostly cats—accidentally fall to the pavement below, sustaining serious injuries or, worse, dying on impact.

Five years earlier, in 1987, while I was an intern at the Animal Medical Center, two of that hospital's surgeons published a first-of-its-kind study[*] in the *Journal of the American Veterinary Medical Association* about what we now call High-Rise Syndrome. When the report initially came out, people were horrified, thinking that the authors were throwing cats out the windows at the hospital. Of course not! At that time, the AMC was also the only emergency hospital open twenty-four hours a day in New York City, so most of these cases went there. They compiled statistics on the 132 cats that were diagnosed over a five-month period with severe injuries sustained due to plummeting from high-rise windows, balconies, and terraces.

Among the important retrospective findings was that a cat's

---

[*] Wayne O. Whitney and Cheryl J. Mehlhaff, "High-Rise Syndrome in Cats," *Journal of the American Veterinary Medical Association* 191, no. 11 (December 1, 1987): 1399–403. Erratum in: *Journal of the American Veterinary Medical Association* 192, no. 4 (February 15, 1988): 542.

survival following a high-rise fall depended on how far it fell. Cats are uniquely equipped with a natural "righting reflex" where they can twist in midair to position themselves feet down during the descent. If a cat falls from six stories or higher, it usually has enough time to right itself and reach "terminal velocity," meaning the cat would stop accelerating. Their bodies would relax and they could land feetfirst. They might survive, but they would likely still suffer fractures, contusions, shock, or ruptured internal organs. What's really fascinating is that a fall from *less* than six stories was much more dangerous because then the cat did not have enough time to right itself and relax before impact, making its injuries more profound. Cats that fell from much higher floors—say, the seventeenth—weren't included in the study, because, sadly, those cats typically died and so weren't brought to a veterinary hospital for care.

As an intern at AMC, I saw at least ten cat High-Rise Syndrome cases, and most of the cats required urgent, costly treatment. Sadly, some who survived the fall had injuries so severe that the only humane thing to do was to euthanize them. These were young, healthy cats—on average, two and a half years old—who were just doing what cats do: exploring, playing, napping on a windowsill, or trying to catch a bird that flew by. All their needless pain and suffering, expensive surgeries, and early deaths could have been prevented by their owners simply closing windows and doors.

The paper was published years before my first visit to King and Queen's whimsical palace in the sky, but it was fresh on my mind because of Steve's recent experience. Just a few weeks before, he was walking on 57th Street when a falling cat landed with an awful *splat* on the sidewalk right in front of him and died on the spot. By pure luck, no person was injured by the falling cat.

Steve immediately went home to hug and kiss Mieskeit and confirm all our windows were tightly closed. It took him a long time to get over witnessing this tragedy.

I'm sorry to be so graphic, but people need to shed the belief that cats are unscathed by precipitous falls. I don't care how many "lives" we think they have, no cat is going to plummet hundreds of feet onto concrete and do well, if they even survive.

As an in-hospital vet, I wouldn't know if my clients had a terrace at their apartment or whether they leave their windows open. I wouldn't even think to ask. But being a *house call* vet, I see for myself the pet hazards that lurk in a client's home. It's a huge advantage to see my patients' home environments, scan for dangers, and advise the client how they can prevent a potential tragedy.

The only problem? Clients who refuse to heed my warnings.

I tried again with Queen Betty and King Don. "Listen to me, please," I urged. "Hundreds of cats die or are seriously injured from high-rise falls every year. I have personally treated too many of them. You can so easily prevent this from happening just by keeping them off the terrace."

"They love it, and I'm not going to stop them," said Don, issuing a royal decree.

I'd only been a house call vet for a few months and so lived in constant fear that my practice would crash and burn at any second. I needed every client I could get, especially ones like Betty and Don who had multiple cats and lots of pet-owning neighbors. They clearly had very strong opinions about how they did things with their animals. I'd resolved "no devil fish on my watch!" but in this instance I lacked the courage of my convictions to push back hard and possibly lose the clients.

To this day, I wish I had. I should have said, "You have a really cute cat. I like him. I want him to live to a ripe old age," or stronger, "If you don't close that door and keep it closed, I cannot be your veterinarian."

Instead, the cat got my tongue, and I didn't say another word about it. I gave Roast Beef and Noodles their exams and vaccinations and continued to see them, despite the open terrace every time I went. Roast Beef became one of my favorite patients. Whenever I worked on him, he did his charming "flop and purr" as soon as I began petting him.

Two years later, on another glorious day in the spring, Betty called me. "Dr. Amy, I have some bad news," she said. I could hear from the timbre in her voice that she'd been crying. "Roast Beef died."

My stomach plunged. "Oh my God. What happened?" I already knew what she was going to say.

"I couldn't find him anywhere, and then our doorman called to say Roast Beef was dead on the sidewalk. He'd fallen off the terrace and landed on Fifth Avenue."

"I'm so very sorry," I said. "He was such a sweet boy. I'll miss him."

My God, what a waste of a life. I was angry and upset, but I held that in during the call. It's not my nature to rub a tragedy in someone's face. The next time I went to see Noodles, the terrace door was finally closed. This family learned its lesson the very hard way.

Thereafter and forever, one of the first things I do when I enter a client's home is to check that the windows, balcony, and terrace doors are closed or screened or open just a crack if they must be at all. And after Roast Beef's death, if a client refuses to take my advice about how to protect their pets from a high-rise fall, I do refuse to be their vet. I have lost clients, but with no regrets since

I did not lose patients. It's sad enough to lose a patient to a disease that medicine can't cure, but I refuse to lose another one to a preventable accident.

There are lots of reasons a client might reject my good advice about protecting their pets from preventable accidents. Sometimes, it might be because they think permissiveness is love, like letting the cats play on the terrace because they want them to be happy. Other times, my message may not get through because of a client's hubris.

When George and I were called to a beautiful duplex on Fifth Avenue, we entered the white marble entryway and took in the elegantly curved staircase that went up to the second floor, and the contemporary and postmodern art that covered every wall. The quantity and quality of the art made sense when I learned that my new client, Jane Tabor, was a dealer of contemporary art.

Jane led George and me though the mid-century modern dining room. We went through the swinging door into a large kitchen with an enormous central island. My entire first apartment wasn't as big as this kitchen.

The granite island was perfect for my exam table, and we neatly unpacked the otoscope, ophthalmoscope, stethoscope, and all of the equipment I would need for a new puppy exam.

I always recommend that a new puppy or kitten be seen as soon as possible when it first comes home to the family. Although not often, I occasionally do find a congenital problem that requires extensive care or that predicts the pet will not live a normal life, and it is better for the client to know this immediately so they can decide whether to keep the puppy or return it to the breeder before they bond too deeply. Most breeders will take the pet back and offer another, but after a few days together the family is too much in love to send the pet back.

Little Lola had been living with Jane and her husband, Richard, for a week, and so far, they reported no problems. Jane brought Lola into the kitchen. Watching her cuddle the puppy, it was obvious that she was already madly in love with Lola.

Please don't let anything be wrong with her, I thought, and began examining the two-pound poodle. As I progressed through my standard protocol, I showed Jane things she should be doing every day to establish the dog's comfort with being touched so she could provide proper hygiene and care, like how to wipe the corners of Lola's eyes to remove the crust that accumulates during sleep, flip her ears over to note their normal color and odor and to wipe away any visible wax, as well as how to brush Lola's teeth.

Then I began my exam of her eyes, ears, teeth, and so on. When I finished all that, I put my stethoscope on and listened to Lola's heart.

Puppy hearts beat very quickly, and I must concentrate to hear the distinct beats and determine if the sounds and rhythm are normal. A heart murmur is an abnormal sound that, like in humans, may indicate the presence of heart disease. The description and location of a murmur are part of the information to determine the cause of the underlying problem.

I listened to Lola's heart and heard a loud *whoosh*ing murmur that is described in veterinary textbooks as the sound of a washing machine, which is associated with a congenital heart defect. If confirmed in Lola, she would need a difficult and expensive heart procedure to try to correct it, but surgical intervention does not guarantee successful repair.

Slowly, I lowered the stethoscope. "I'm afraid I've found something I don't want to hear in a young puppy," I said to Jane. Her eyes widened. "Lola has a heart murmur. This type is associated with a congenital heart defect. To know exactly what we're dealing with, Lola needs to see a veterinary cardiologist and have an echocardiogram."

"Is this serious?" asked Jane, already scared and shaky.

I owed it to her to be honest. "It could be serious, but I won't know until she's had the echo."

She burst into tears. "Is Lola going to die?"

"I need more information, and once we have it, I will be able to explain the problem and what the possible treatment options are."

Jane was full-on sobbing now. She put her hands over her face and ran out of the room with the puppy.

I looked at George, who said, "You had to tell her."

Of course I did. The whole point of doing the exam was to gather information to provide to the owner about their new pet's health, and that was what I'd done. But I still felt terrible that I'd upset her so. This case might not be so bad, but I needed the echocardiogram results to be sure. I waited ten minutes, and since I didn't know if Jane was coming back, I said to George, "Let's start packing up. I'll call her later with the name of a cardiologist."

George and I loaded up the last of our equipment just as a large man punched through the kitchen's swinging doors and burst into the room. He was over six feet, gray-haired, red-faced, and was coming in hot. I took a step back. He stuck his finger in my face and screamed at me, "How *dare* you diagnose my dog with a fatal congenital heart defect! How *dare* you say she's going to die!"

"I didn't say . . ."

"What do *you* know about cardiology? What do *you* know about the heart?" He was screaming so loud it hurt my ears, and some of his spittle landed on my cheek.

George stood next to me and put his hand on my shoulder. "Sir,

Dr. Attas hasn't yet diagnosed your dog. She heard an abnormality and recommended an echocardiogram."

I appreciated his support. This man was almost more frightening than Rocky the rottweiler with a corneal ulcer.

"You don't know *anything* about cardiology," he raved. "I know more than you ever will. I invented the first heart valve. You are a terrible veterinarian with a god-awful bedside manner. My wife is crying her eyes out because you just told her the dog is as good as dead."

"Again, sir, I did *not* say that. I heard a murmur, and it's important Lola have an echocardiogram to find out what's going on."

"Don't tell me about echocardiograms! I know *everything* about echocardiograms! *I invented the first damn artificial heart valve!*"

I couldn't find the words to calm down this unhinged man because my own heart was pounding so loudly in my chest. I might need one of his artificial valves before this was over. If he invented cardiac medical devices, then he knew a lot about the heart, and he'd probably dissected hundreds of human cadaver hearts in his day. But I had listened to a thousand live dogs' hearts and absolutely knew a murmur when I heard one. Did he have *veterinary* training? Had *he* listened to Lola's heart?

None of that mattered. His wife broke down because of what I told her. I was the cause of *that*—but not his puppy's medical problem.

"Just get the hell out of my house!" he commanded.

He didn't have to ask us twice. We were gone in seconds. In the elevator, I asked George, "Am I crazy? I thought I was sensitive but straight with the client."

"You absolutely were! This is a case of killing the messenger," he reassured me.

Still, I had to wonder if I could have handled it better.

That afternoon, I left a message on their answering machine with the name and number of a veterinary cardiologist. Although no one called me back, as the referring doctor I did hear from the cardiologist a few days later that he'd seen Lola and diagnosed her as I suspected, with a serious congenital heart defect. At that point, I was no longer Lola's vet, and it wasn't appropriate for me to remain in the loop. I had no idea whether they decided to repair the defect or return the puppy to the breeder. I was sad to hear the extent of Lola's heart condition but felt gratified that my detection of the murmur had been confirmed.

Flash forward ten years. Steve and I went to a Broadway play with our dear friends Vanessa and James. During intermission, we went to the lobby to get a drink. Vanessa and James apparently ran into some of their own friends, and I watched them exchange hugs and kisses. They called us over to introduce us, and I nearly choked on my seltzer when I saw that their friends were Jane and Richard Tabor.

They smiled placidly at me, thankfully without a glimmer of recognition.

While the four of them chatted away, I pinched Steve on the leg. He jerked his head and gave me a look to say, "What?"

I maneuvered him a few feet to the side and whispered, "That's the heart valve guy."

It took a second for him to remember. "The one who screamed at you?"

"They don't recognize me at all."

After the show, Steve and I went to dinner with Vanessa and James, and I told them the story about Richard Tabor's meltdown. James said, "They *did* have a dog that died young from heart disease. I guess that was around ten years ago. I love the guy, but he has a reputation for being a total jerk."

I concurred.

Flash forward fifteen more years. Carida took a call from one Jane Tabor, at the same Fifth Avenue address we had in our system. Mrs. Tabor asked, "I heard about your house call service from a friend. Are you taking new clients?"

She said, "We're taking new clients" . . . *and old ones,* she thought, as she noted their earlier records. Carida scheduled a wellness check for their brand-new toy poodle puppy. History was repeating itself. This time, when I arrived at the same duplex with the same glorious art on the walls, I introduced myself to Jane as if we'd never met. She either genuinely didn't remember me or was playing along. The good news was that their new puppy was totally healthy.

Before I left, Richard Tabor came through those swinging doors and smiled placidly at me. He was in his late eighties by then, and time had apparently mellowed him. He was sweet as could be.

I go to their apartment often these days, and neither they nor I have ever mentioned that first tempestuous visit, much less Mr. Tabor's outburst. He's never said to me, "You were right about Lola, and I was out of line." But that happened so long ago, I no longer needed an apology. And Jane has turned out to be a loyal, wonderful client who takes every piece of advice I give her.

The Franklins, a middle-aged couple who lived on East 94th Street and Madison Avenue, were borderline pet hoarders. Every six months, they called me to say they'd adopted yet another dog or cat. Their menagerie peaked at *eight* animals. That was a lot of fur to vacuum up in a two-bedroom apartment.

Every time this couple got a pet, Mrs. Franklin proclaimed he or she was the "love of my life!" And the Franklins lived up to that, doting on their animals, pampering them, showering them with as much love and attention as they'd show to a human child if they had one.

George and I showed up for our monthly visit for Sushi, an elderly, chronically constipated Siamese cat, and found a very excited Mrs. Franklin.

"I couldn't wait to tell you both, a miracle has happened!" she said. "My husband and I have been trying to have a baby for nearly twenty years, and after all this time, I'm finally pregnant!"

"Congratulations!" I said. "I'm so happy for you!"

"Thank you! The baby is healthy, and I'm doing great. We can't wait to welcome her into our lives in a few months. But we do have one problem."

"How can I help?" I asked.

"We need to get rid of all our animals," she said. "I hope you can find homes for them."

What?! You can't be a pet hoarder one day and the next just sweep them out of your house!

"No, no, that's not necessary," I said. "Ninety percent of the homes I go to are families with children and pets. It's wonderful for kids to grow up with animals."

She insisted, "We're not going to do that. We don't want animals near our baby."

I tried one more time. "I'm the first person to say, 'Don't leave your baby unattended with an animal.' But things you might have heard—like cats smothering babies—are urban myths. If you're careful and smart, your baby and pets will be fine together, and each will love the other."

But Mrs. Franklin just did not want to hear it. "If you're not going to give them away for us, we're simply going to take them to the ASPCA and have them put to sleep."

Now I was really stunned. I've seen and heard some shocking things in my life as vet. But this floored me. Every single one of her pets was "the absolute love of my life!" And now she just casually talked about euthanizing them. All of them.

I blurted, "I'll take them all," having no plan other than to somehow save these innocent lives.

Within two weeks, I found homes for all eight pets, even the constipated Siamese. George had always loved their black-and-white cat Gato, named after the Argentinian jazz saxophonist, so he adopted him.

Once the last animal was rehomed, I never spoke to the Franklins again. If they called me today to say, "We adopted a cat and she's the love of my life!" I'd politely end the call.

It is unconscionable that anyone would threaten to put down healthy animals to make their lives more convenient. If someone accumulates animals to fill their home and heart, that person has a moral obligation, an unbreakable contract, to care for those innocent creatures for their entire lives. I'll say it again: *for their entire lives*. That is what it means to be a good parent, for a child or for a fur baby. That is what it means to be human.

There *was* a time when I lost my cool with a client over her bad behavior.

The young family lived on Park Avenue in a building I went to often because I had other clients there as well. Joyce Gordon, a thirtysomething mom with two small children, had an adorable, rambunctious Yorkie named Zoe. I met Zoe when she arrived as a puppy and did her puppy shots, arranged her spay, and did her annual exams. Zoe was the center of attention in that family.

When Zoe was around seven, the Gordons brought in a pair of kittens. Suddenly, Zoe was less interesting to the family. They seemed to have transferred all the affection to the new kittens. Whenever Carida and I went to their house to examine the pair, it was heartbreaking to see Zoe ignored. The poor dog could be found sitting alone in another room when previously she was in the middle of everything.

A year later, Mrs. Gordon called me to say, "We're thinking of giving up Zoe. The doorman loves her. What do you think of the idea?"

I thought it was lousy.

On the other hand, I knew how much the doorman loved Zoe because he told me every time I came to the building. But I was concerned because Zoe had Cushing's disease, a common disorder in aging small-breed dogs, caused by a tiny tumor in the pituitary gland of the brain. The presence of the tumor itself isn't a problem. But it produces a hormone that triggers the adrenal glands to put out extra cortisone. As a result, Cushing's dogs drink a lot of water and may urinate in the house. Over time they lose their fur and develop skin conditions, their livers become enlarged giving them potbellies, and the disease predisposes them to other medical issues. These signs are preventable with daily medication, and Zoe's symptoms were well controlled.

Giving away the family's adult dog? What about the trauma Zoe might suffer being suddenly ripped from her family? But I addressed only the practical aspects. "As she gets older, her Cushing's may cause other problems. Is Jose financially equipped to take on a dog with her issues?"

"Not a problem," she replied quickly. "I already thought of that.

We'll take care of the vet bills as long as she lives." Such planning made it seem as if she were a little too eager for Zoe to leave.

Mrs. Gordon was a stay-at-home mom, and her husband worked on Wall Street and made gazillions of dollars. It was no hardship for them to pay for Zoe's lifetime medical care, which they would have done anyway if she stayed with them.

"Sounds like you already have a plan," I said. Although I couldn't understand a family's giving up their little dog they had loved for years, if they had already made this decision then Jose was a perfect choice.

I don't judge people who need to rehome pets because, say, a family member develops an allergy or they are moving far away or for any number of true and good reasons. I've happily helped clients rehome pets scores of times. But Mrs. Gordon wanted to give away a dog who, at one point, had been the center of her family's universe just because she lost interest when new pets arrived. If you had a child, would you suddenly stop caring about them when you had a second child?

I didn't bother trying to figure out how Mrs. Gordon could be so cavalier with the life of an animal that plainly loved her family so much. But, then again, without question, at this point Zoe would be better off with someone who actually wanted her.

Over the next few years, Jose, who lived in Queens, brought Zoe to work with him on the days I came to give her a checkup. I treated her various problems in the basement of the Park Avenue building in the doormen's break room. Zoe did eventually develop diabetes, and Jose managed the twice-daily insulin injections perfectly. "I just love this dog, Doc," Jose always told me. "I'm so glad to have her, I would do anything for her." I was happy for both Zoe and the doorman that things were working out so well.

One Monday, I showed up at the building to see another

family's pet. As I walked in, Jose asked, "Doc, can I talk to you for a second?"

"Of course."

"Zoe wasn't at all well over the weekend. She seemed to be in a lot of pain, so I took her to the emergency vet near my place in Queens. They examined her and took X-rays and found a large stone in her bladder. She needs to have surgery as soon as possible."

"We knew something like this could happen because of Zoe's diabetes," I replied. "I'll make a call and set up the surgery right away."

Jose's eyes filled with tears as he continued. "The problem is, I told Mrs. Gordon what was happening, and she said, 'I think I've fulfilled my requirements for Zoe with you. You should consider her your own dog from now on.' Those were her exact words."

I was stunned. The surgery alone would cost over two thousand dollars, a big chunk of Jose's annual salary—and far less than what Mrs. Gordon spends on a new handbag.

I was outraged. With fingers of fury, I dialed her right then and there, and said, "I was shocked when I heard from your doorman that you are reneging on your promise to cover Zoe's bills. He loves her more than anything. You gave Zoe to him, and he took her on knowing that although he couldn't afford her care, *you promised him* you would pay her vet bills. And now in the last years of her life, when her care is more expensive, you're going back on your promise?!" I took a deep breath and added, "Reneging on Jose is really a shitty thing to do."

Yes. I said "shitty."

I wanted her to feel guilty about breaking her promise to someone in an unequal situation who had relied on her commitment of support and would likely not have been able to adopt Zoe otherwise. I wouldn't have put it past her to try to make trouble for Jose after he confided in me, but he was protected by the strong NYC doorman's union. His job was not at risk—but now Zoe was.

"Dr. Amy, this isn't your business," she said with icy calm. "Your services are no longer required."

I replied angrily, "You can't fire me. I'm firing you!"

If that was how she treated the man who came to her rescue and took in her dog when she wanted to toss it out, I didn't want anything more to do with her. Mrs. Gordon didn't seem to care how disgusted I was with her or that her doorman actually had to reach into his retirement savings to pay for Zoe's surgery. She simply did what she wanted to do. And still, every day, Jose opened the door for her and smiled when she walked through because he was the better person in every sense that mattered.

Zoe was as devoted to Jose as he was to her. I could always see in her eyes how much she loved him in a way I never saw her express when she belonged to Mrs. Gordon. Dogs really are the best judges of character. Though in this case, I wasn't far behind.

Rudeness, I've learned, is a thin mask for deeper feelings. When people are upset about the well-being of their pets, they might take out their fear and anxiety on others, namely, me and my staff. The trigger is usually that a client doesn't get exactly what they want. Often that involves an appointment, as scheduling is one of the hardest jobs for the City Pets office team because it's hard to predict how much time a typical call will take. There are always issues.

Sometimes we arrive at a call as scheduled, but the building may have no elevator and we haven't factored in the time needed to trudge up the stairwell to the fifth floor carrying our equipment. Or we're slowed down when a client asks us to look at their other pets ("After all, you're here"). Often, it's Manhattan traffic, which can be at a standstill at any time . . . such as when the UN General Assembly opens or there's an unannounced street closure for construction. And sometimes, it's just a lot of sick pets that need our unscheduled attention.

It was a combination of factors that came into play one harried day, and I sent Carida, who was at the office, an email that said I had no room for any add-on calls. It was already after noon and I'd gotten through only a third of the day's scheduled calls.

A few minutes later, Peter, a longtime client we hadn't seen in years, called the office to make an appointment. Carida was delighted to hear from him. We'd cared for two of his elderly cats, Rigoletto and Salome, until they passed about five years prior.

He remembered her fondly, too. After they chatted for a few minutes, he said, "Carida, I need to make an appointment for my cat, Carmen. You guys haven't seen her before."

Even though I told her I was fully booked, Carida liked him, so she checked the schedule anyway, thinking maybe she could move some things around. Seeing it was not possible, she said, "We're all booked for today, but Dr. Amy can come tomorrow afternoon."

Without objection, he booked the slot. A few minutes later, he sent her a video of Carmen. Carida forwarded it to me immediately. "Take a look at this cat. I think you need to see her today."

The video showed Carmen, an adult cat, sitting awkwardly on the floor breathing rapidly with her mouth open. Nothing good causes a cat to breathe with their mouth open. Cats don't pant like dogs do, and open-mouthed breathing can be a sign of cardiac or respiratory illness, or a number of other things, all bad.

I texted right back, "Agreed, she can't wait until tomorrow. Call Peter. I will be there as soon possible."

Carida called Peter but had to leave a voicemail message saying, "Call me back to confirm that you are at home and that Dr. Amy can come now." She was thinking that since he didn't answer, he might have already taken Carmen to the emergency room.

When he called back a minute later, his tone was angry. "Why did you tell me you couldn't see Carmen until tomorrow and now she could be seen today? My cat is really sick and you turned me away!"

"You didn't tell me your cat was sick," she replied, annoyed. "You should have told me she was sick. We always find a way to fit in sick patients."

If we don't have an open time for a sick pet, we make one by going through the schedule and finding a patient that perhaps is getting a routine checkup or a vaccination, which can wait a day or two. But a patient having difficulty breathing needs to be seen right away.

"Why are you yelling at me?" he yelled at Carida, really riled up now.

She stared at the phone, dumbfounded. "I'm not yelling at you, sir. Do you want Dr. Amy to come over?"

"Yes!" he barked, and slammed the phone down.

Jeanine was with me for our visit to Carmen and Peter. He still lived in the same one-bedroom in Chelsea that he shared with his husband, John. As soon as we walked in, I remembered the place. Nothing had changed. I was again impressed by the apartment's neatness. Everything—the furniture, rugs, stainless steel appliances—looked brand-new. The open bookcases held perfectly arranged books by size and color.

I quickly asked Peter my standard questions and learned that he and John had adopted Carmen as a spayed kitten five and a half years ago.

"Has she had her vaccinations?" I asked.

"I don't think so," he said.

"Has she been tested for feline leukemia, feline immunodeficiency virus, or *Bartonella henselae*?" All three of these conditions increased her risk for disease. On a new kitten exam, I did blood tests for all of them.

"I don't think so, no," he said.

"Can I take a look at her medical records?" I asked.

"We don't have any. We haven't taken her to a vet since we adopted her."

"Five and a half years ago?" I asked incredulously.

"Correct."

Jeanine's mouth dropped open. She could not hide her concern, and I shared it. Imagine not taking your child to a doctor in five years. Peter meticulously cared for his possessions, but he didn't do even the bare minimum to care for his cat's health. I buried my irritation in order to do my job.

"Where is Carmen now?" I asked.

He brought us into the bedroom, and there I found a gray tabby sitting up on a wide windowsill on a pillow.

He said, "She been holding her mouth open since yesterday and hasn't eaten since then."

Although I initially feared that the open mouth was related to a breathing problem, that was not the case. Thick saliva tinged with blood and a very foul odor emanated from Carmen's mouth. I put on my headlamp and Jeanine gently held Carmen so I could get a good look in her mouth. Her breath smelled like rotting meat. Her gums were swollen and bleeding. I couldn't find many of her teeth because they had literally disintegrated, and portions of their roots were exposed. No wonder Carmen wasn't eating and was holding her mouth open—she was in remarkable pain.

"Peter, come closer. I need you to see what's going on here," I said. I pointed out the inflammation of her gums. He crinkled his nose as he smelled the rot and looked away when I opened her mouth and he saw the bleeding tissue.

"The foul odor is coming from the infection in her mouth. Her abnormal breathing is like this because *she is in pain*. This has been going on for a while, and now her pain is just more than she can handle."

"Do you think it would've made a difference if we caught it earlier?" he asked.

Jeanine swallowed a groan. I nearly snapped, *"What did I just say?"* but didn't.

Instead, I nodded and said, "Yes. It might even have started when she was a kitten. If caught earlier, we would have known about the dental disease and taken preventive measures, like teaching you how to do proper oral hygiene for her."

I remained nonjudgmental with Peter. It wouldn't help Carmen to make him feel more horrible, but I was angry about his neglect.

To deal with the infection, I gave Carmen an injection of Convenia, a long-lasting antibiotic that is much more convenient for clients than giving pills, especially when their pet's mouth is hurting. I also gave her an injection for her pain.

"This injection is not going to solve the problem," I said. "She needs to have dental work as soon as possible. She will be under general anesthesia. Her mouth will be assessed by X-ray and all the diseased teeth and roots will be extracted. Right now, the diseased teeth are painful, and once they are out, the pain will be gone."

Jeanine gently laid Carmen on her side and I took the blood tests needed for her upcoming procedure, including tests for all the diseases that might explain why a young cat had such significant oral cavity issues.

I further explained that because Carmen had never been vaccinated for feline distemper or rabies, it would be best to do that before her hospitalization. "But not today, because of her infection," I said. "She'll need a follow-up antibiotic shot in two weeks, and I can take care of her missing vaccines when I return. I am sure she will be feeling better by then. Don't forget to call the office to schedule that."

Every single test and vaccine I recommended would have been done already if I, or any vet, had been seeing this cat since kittenhood. Jeanine and I took the samples and left, keeping our anger to ourselves and knowing that Carmen would start to feel a little better soon.

Two days later, Peter called the office to report that Carmen was eating and keeping her mouth closed. Carida emailed the invoice, and the next day charged the credit card on file as is our practice. Three days later, the bank reported that the credit card charge was reversed. I assumed it was some kind of glitch.

After two weeks without contact to schedule our visit, I called Peter from the back seat of the car while on my way to my next house call. "You're at the two-week point," I said. "The infection is going to come back if we don't give her another injection. And we really need to schedule your cat's dental. Oh, and do you know why the charges on your credit card were reversed?"

Peter replied angrily, "I'm not having you come back. I never want to see you again. Your receptionist was rude to me and lied about there not being any appointments, and I'm not paying this bill."

"I don't understand."

"What kind of practice do you run? Your assistant yelled at me."

Seriously? He was stewing about that phone call? He was plainly projecting his bad behavior onto Carida. *He* was the one who yelled. Frankly, he should feel shame—not because of anything we did, but because not only was he rude to my staff but because he had neglected Carmen's health. And now he was yelling *at me*.

"If you felt uncomfortable about what my assistant said to you, why did you book the appointment with me and allow us to incur all of these expenses?" I asked. "You could have gone elsewhere."

He hung up on me.

Immediately, I called his husband, John, and said, "I just spoke to Peter, and he gave me an earful and is refusing to pay our bill."

John knew the whole saga, and said, "He's overreacting, and I can't talk any sense into him. I think he feels guilty about what happened to Carmen. Don't worry, I'll take care of the bill." He gave me a new credit card number, and that was that. We never heard from this family again. To this day, I hope Carmen got her vaccines and dental procedure.

The top-line atrocious behavior was Peter's neglect of his cat's health to the point that she was in agonizing pain. He knew better, having had cats in the past. Carmen's decline could have been arrested if he'd just taken her to a vet as soon as he noticed her foul breath—or at any point in the last few years for that matter. And there was simply no excuse for ignoring Carmen's vaccines when he first adopted her.

It was too difficult for him to accept his own guilt and shame, so he put it on us. I tried not to show anger, and I hope I succeeded. But honestly, my overriding emotion throughout was sadness for this cat who suffered because of her owner's negligence.

CHAPTER 9

Standout Days

Whatcould be better than making a pet feel better? Truly almost nothing. But being a *house call* vet also puts me in standout situations that add to the fun and richness of my job.

Some days are joyous, such as when my client's eight-year-old daughter watches me examine their wheaten terrier with laser-like focus and then announces her intention to become a vet. And years later she does! (Of course, I lose her parents as my clients when she graduates and has her own practice.)

And some days are genuinely funny. And some days you just can't make this stuff up.

Henry, an accountant, lived in a third-floor walk-up apartment on First Avenue. It was not an easy place for us to make house calls as the apartment was small, and his kitchen was neither clean nor well-lit. The linoleum countertop where I wanted to place my patient was tacky from a thin layer of grease. The smell of burned cooking oil was always in the air, and I smelled from it after we left.

George and I came here often because Henry's cocker spaniel, Ruby, constantly got into trouble. Just a month before, Ruby clawed open the faux-wood-paneled kitchen cabinet door to get to her food bag. She ate almost her full weight in kibble, and I had to make her vomit because she was so bloated, she could barely move.

She suffered the indignity graciously because she was such a sweet dog. And cute, too. Her tawny fur was a perfect match for the "hair" on top of Henry's own head, but hers was real. You would think if someone was vain enough to hide his baldness, he'd get a toupee that looked at least real-*ish*. But Henry didn't have a lot of style. He wore plaid polyester blazers, trousers with an overworn shine, his belt hitched three inches too high, and a toupee that looked, well, ridiculous.

That day, Ruby was dragging her rear on the wall-to-wall beige carpet. "Does she have worms?" he asked when I arrived. "She ate something weird on the street the other day."

Every dog and cat, male and female, has anal glands located at the five and seven o'clock positions inside the opening of their rectum. These glands fill with a fetid material that they release when stressed, like skunks famously do. In the wild, stressed animals squirt their rancid load as a warning to their own kind of possible danger.

While domestic animals don't roam the forest and their lives are relatively cushy, their anal glands fill up anyway, and they are emptied when the animal grooms itself or when the gland gets compressed during the passing of a large bowel movement. A signal that the gland is full and that the animal is unable to empty it themselves is the funny Charlie Chaplin scoot along the floor they do to rub the gland to empty it. If successful, you will know; there will be a noxious smell on your carpet. Most likely, your pet will lick it up; if not, Purell works.

Birds gotta fly. Fish gotta swim. Dogs gotta lick anal fluid off the rug. It's kind of gross, but it's their nature.

But if the glands remain clogged, the situation goes from funny to frightening, fast. Clogged glands can turn into abscesses. When this happens, the infected glands need to be drained and the patient put on antibiotics.

I examined Ruby and concluded that her glands were full and clogged and had to be emptied manually, as she was on her way to developing an abscess. Today's visit should prevent the infection from happening. It's not the most glamorous procedure I do, but it is important. With a well-lubricated glove on, I insert my index finger into the patient's rectum. My thumb remains on the outside, and then using both fingers, I milk the gland toward its opening until about a tablespoon or more of the trapped, stinky gunk comes out.

I began to do this for Ruby and warned Henry, "I'm going to recommend you stand way back."

Most clients leave the room for this procedure, but not Henry. He moved in even closer and was hovering right at my shoulder, so close that I could smell his toupee tonic, which wasn't pleasant.

"You're blocking my light," I said. There wasn't enough as it was.

"Sorry," he said, but only moved an inch.

Prep work completed, it was time to insert my finger and start expressing the gland's material. It took only a few motions to feel that Ruby was quite full and clogged.

George spoke softly to Ruby while I carried on. And Henry kept inching closer to me to get a good view. "You *really do* need to back up," I warned him again. He didn't.

I applied a bit more pressure to the gland, and that did it. A gush of bloody, foul-smelling butt juice squirted out . . . and landed right on top of Henry's toupee.

"Whoa!" he screamed, and stumbled backward. "That's horrible!"

The smell is indeed one of a kind, like skunk meets rotten fish. It's hard to get the stink out of clothes, and I couldn't begin to imagine how to get it out of a toupee. This time, not a drop landed on me.

Ruby was immediately relieved and wagged her tail. Henry did not.

We left and stifled our laughter walking back down the three flights to the street knowing that voices carry in stairwells. Once we hit the street, we couldn't help cracking up.

George said, "Look at the bright side. Now he'll have to get a new toupee."

I was Ruby's vet for her entire life. Henry never crowded me again. His subsequent toupees were no improvement.

One evening that started out the wrong way wound up enormously satisfying because I am a house call vet.

Le Cirque, a French restaurant and famed New York institution, had recently moved to its new location in the Palace Hotel on Madison Avenue, and the whole City was desperate to get a reservation. One of Steve's business associates knew Sirio Maccioni, the owner, and he managed to get us a reservation. Since Steve's associate made the reservation directly with Sirio himself, we assumed we'd be treated well.

We arrived at the restaurant, beautifully dressed and excited. Sirio himself was at the door when we walked in, heard our name, looked at us—and turned his head away and ignored us. The maître d' then kept us waiting for half an hour before he took us to our table. Things did not get better. He led us through the all-important see-and-be-seen front room, then the middle room for B-listers, and finally to our table way in the back, all by itself and next to the bathroom. It was the single worst table in the restaurant.

This was going to be a very expensive dinner, and no matter how good the food was, being seated right next to the bathroom was unacceptable. Steve told him that we would not sit there, and the maître d' sniffed impatiently. "I am sorry, sir. We're fully booked. I won't have another table for at least an hour."

Even though my stomach was grumbling with hunger, Steve said, "We will wait." The maître d' was very put out by this, and hurriedly led us back to the waiting area. As he marched us through the front room, we passed by a large round center table—truly the best in the house—with six diners.

I thought, *Who do you have to know—or be—to sit there?*

Just as we were skirting the table, one of its occupants exclaimed in my direction, "Dr. Amy! Dr. Amy! Oh my God, you'll never believe this, but *we were just talking about you!*"

Seated at the table were clients of mine in the newspaper business. One owned *The New York Observer* and the other was the family that owned *The Washington Post*. And with them were their newspapers' restaurant critics. Apparently, when media elite dine at the hottest restaurant in town, they talk about their vets.

The rude maître d' was stunned by their recognition of me, and he was now staring at us with a horror that said he might have just been disrespectful to someone important after all.

Sirio then entered the fray as he rushed over to us immediately. He panted, "I'm so sorry for the confusion. Your table is ready now."

He then escorted us to the *second best* table in the restaurant, in the main room and just a few feet from my clients. Throughout the evening, extra treats from the kitchen kept magically appearing on our table. We got VIP treatment from that moment on—but only because my famous clients happened to be there that night to validate me.

Two days later, I went to Joan Rivers's apartment to see Spike, and Kevin, her house manager asked me, "So how was your dinner at Le Cirque?"

"What? How did you know I was there?"

"I read the restaurant review in *The New York Observer*."

The vet—*me!*—was in the review.

We never returned to Le Cirque because of the way they treated us before the VIP dust floated onto us from my clients. Just like the maître d', I provide customer service, too, and I would never treat any client with anything but courtesy, kindness, and patience, whether they were a Master of the Universe or Gail the Hoarder. Everybody deserves that same level of respect, though apparently not at Le Cirque.

The food, however, was excellent.

Normally, I like nothing better than examining a healthy puppy with their furry little faces and warm, furry, wiggly little bodies. But this puppy visit was not going to be fun. It was a house call to Mrs. Goldschmidt, and she presented me with a box of twelve two-day-old Irish setter pups. The puppies each needed a thorough checkup and to have their two front dewclaws removed. This was going to take me all day.

Dewclaws are odd little lumps of skin with a nail attached located at the base of the forearm. They are vestigial thumbs that serve no purpose, and they cause problems. Dewclaws get caught on brush when a dog is outside and on fabric when inside, and they occasionally get accidentally ripped off altogether. It's generally agreed in veterinary medicine that it is best to remove them when a puppy is a newborn to avoid such future problems.

In theory, removing a dewclaw is a minor procedure. A small incision to remove it, and one stitch to close it up. It shouldn't take more than fifteen seconds. In reality, it takes forever because puppies do not stay still. When I ask them politely to stop moving long enough so I can do their surgical procedure, they don't listen. And these Irish setter pups were already wriggling like worms.

While I set up my instruments and prepared myself for the work ahead, a memory popped into my head. It was of the rabbi who recently performed the circumcision on my brother's newborn son. My nephew was crying and flailing about during the prayers leading to the procedure. I wondered how the rabbi was going to perform this delicate procedure on a very sensitive part of the thrashing baby's anatomy. If the baby moved at just the wrong moment, dire consequences would remain with him for the rest of his life!

I remember noticing that before the rabbi began his surgical procedure, he dipped a napkin into a glass of wine that he'd blessed. Then he explained to the attendees that the baby needed to share the "ceremonial" wine, and he put the end of the purple-soaked napkin into the baby's mouth. Within seconds of starting to suckle on the napkin, the baby stopped wiggling, and the rabbi got to work on a quiescent patient. He had used the blessed wine as an anesthetic.

The subconscious mind is remarkable. By sending me this memory at that moment, I thought of a solution to my current problem. Could the wine trick work with puppies, too?

I turned to Mrs. Goldschmidt, and asked, "Do you have any sweet wine in the house?"

"*Really*, Dr. Amy?" she asked wide-eyed. Her expression killed me. She seemed to think I was asking to have a glass of wine in the middle of the day for my nerves before I did a surgical procedure.

But with faith in me, she said, "Yes, I do have some. Be right back." She went into the kitchen and came back with a bottle and a wineglass, no further questions.

I poured some wine into the glass and immersed the end of a Q-tip into it. I picked up the first puppy and put the wine-soaked Q-tip into his mouth. Just like my baby nephew, the puppy began to suckle it and within seconds, he was asleep. I didn't hesitate. I completed the dewclaw removal, and this time, it really did take just fifteen seconds! As I admired my work, the puppy woke and began to wriggle again. I placed him in the box so he could nurse on his mother.

The other eleven puppies seemed to line up to get the Q-tip delivery of a sweet wine treat. I did the remaining surgeries in record time.

I was just finishing the last one when Mrs. Goldschmidt left the room and came back with *two* wineglasses.

"That was like heaven to watch, Dr. Amy. You deserve a toast."

I laughed as she poured us each a glass of wine. She raised hers and said, "To their health." We clinked and drank to the health of the puppies. I made a mental note to add a tiny glass of wine to my traveling medical supply suitcase, though I declined my nurse's suggestion to write this up for a veterinary journal.

The whole thing went very well, in fact, so much better than my nephew's circumcision. I'll confess that as I watched the rabbi begin that process on my nephew, I fainted right to the floor. Apparently, I never did get fully over that fainting problem.

The summer of 1995 was one of the hottest on record in New York. And yet, my new driver, Omar, refused to turn on the AC.

"Doc, the AC won't work unless I get more Freon, and that costs four hundred bucks," he said.

George snapped, "It's always something with you and this car."

These two never got along. But George was right. Omar did have a tendency to ask me to pay for expensive repairs to his car. But the last thing anyone needed was a heated argument. We were already melting. I wrote Omar a check and asked him to deal with it right away.

A week later, the heat still unbearable, the AC still out, we drove to our first stop of the day at the home of Mary Catherine, one half of the pair we called "the Sisters."

She and her sister, Peggy Sue, were both longtime clients. Neither had ever married, both were in their mid-sixties. Mary Catherine lived on East 21st Street in a brownstone that overlooked Gramercy Park. Peggy Sue lived on East 88th Street in a similar building down the street from Central Park. The apartments and their décor were nearly identical, like their wardrobes. Even their cats were matching. Each Sister had two, one white tabby and one gray tabby each. The cats were so similar I usually got their names confused.

Mary Catherine had called us because her tabby was having a little trouble breathing. His eyes and nose were running, and he was sneezing all the time. He was a pretty fat cat, and he wasn't eating as much as usual. I suspected he had an upper respiratory infection, and we scheduled an appointment for that day.

After a scorching ride downtown, the doorman let us into Mary Catherine's apartment and we examined Charlie. Despite the runny nose and sneezing, all else was fine. I called Mary Catherine and said he just had a cold, like people get. "It's probably a good idea to put out the smelliest cat food you can find, and his appetite will come back. If he's not better in a few days, call me."

I wasn't surprised to get a call from sister Peggy Sue the next day. It seemed inevitable that if one of their cats had a cold, the other's would, too. Bobby had a runny nose and trouble breathing. Peggy Sue tried the smelly food trick I gave Mary Catherine with her cat, but he still wouldn't eat.

After another car-sauna drive uptown, George and I arrived at Peggy Sue's soaked in sweat and went up to her apartment to examine Bobby. We couldn't find him. We searched low and high for half an hour, increasingly frustrated and concerned.

"I'm not going to lie," said George as he plunked down on the couch. "I'm loving the air-conditioning."

It was wonderful, but there was no time to relax. After a room-to-room search, I finally found Bobby scrunched behind the toilet tank. His breathing was dramatically labored. This was no cold. Bobby needed to get to the animal hospital immediately. George found the cat carrier in the front hall closet, and we rushed Bobby back down to the street.

Omar was standing in the shade of the building's awning, chatting with the doorman.

George and I piled into the car, and I yelled to Omar, "We have to get to the hospital right away!" Not understanding my urgency, Omar meandered into the driver's seat and we headed for the Center for Veterinary Care a few blocks away. It should have taken no more than several minutes, but the traffic was monstrous. We crawled down Second Avenue and then came to a complete standstill. As the temperature in the car rose, Bobby's breathing worsened. The poor cat was running out of time.

"For God's sake, crank the air-conditioning!" I screamed.

Omar said, "I'm sorry, Doc. I never got the Freon."

George turned to him and had some choice words for Omar. They started yelling at each other, which didn't help one bit.

Without a word to either one of them, I threw the door open, got out of the car, grabbed the cat carrier, and started running down Second Avenue in the middle of the stopped traffic. The bulky cat carrier swinging at my hip as I ran, I dodged and weaved across two lanes of cars, leaped onto the sidewalk, zigzagged through crowds, and then bolted hard right on East 75th Street toward the hospital.

As soon as I burst through the doors, I yelled, "I need oxygen, *stat!*" to the ER nurse.

Someone took the cat carrier out of my hand, and Bobby was rushed into an oxygen cage where he soon began to breathe a bit more normally. I doubled over, hands on my knees, chest heaving and sweat pouring down my front and my back.

When I looked up, I noticed that some of the hospital staffers were gathered around, laughing at me.

"What's so funny?" I wheezed, still catching my breath.

Una, the hospital manager, said, "We didn't know if the O_2 was for you or your patient!"

Look-alike cats belonging to identical sisters had identical symptoms, but their conditions couldn't have been more different. One cat had the sniffles, while the other had a potentially fatal heart condition.

Both cats survived the day, but Omar's employment with City Pets didn't.

CHAPTER 10

Bold-Faced Names

Some of the best parts of my job are meeting incredible people, being in places I'd never otherwise be, or having one-of-a-kind experiences.

For instance, several years into the practice, a woman called. "I got your number from a friend," she said, "and I hope you can help us. We just got a new puppy. She's lethargic and won't stop coughing."

Healthy puppies run, chew table legs, and destroy expensive loafers. So I was concerned about the opposite: a sleepy, coughing puppy.

The client gave me her address, which was conveniently just a few blocks from my next appointment. "I'll be there in the next hour," I told her, happy that I could provide such great service.

"Thank you! My name is Janet Jones. Tell the doorman and he'll let you right up," she said. I knew that she was a famous actress but there was something else about her that I couldn't recall. As soon as I walked in to the apartment and saw the hockey sticks by the door and the large, framed jersey on the wall, I remembered that Janet Jones was married to the greatest hockey player of all time, Wayne Gretzky, who was then playing for the New York Rangers. My husband and I are avid hockey fans and in fact had season tickets to the Rangers. *Oh boy, Steve is going to be jealous!*

Just then, Gretzky himself walked into the entrance hallway with an adorable toy poodle puppy in his arms. She immediately began hacking.

"Liberty has been coughing like this since we brought her home," Gretzky said. "But it's much worse at night. She sleeps in our bedroom, and for the past three nights she's been up coughing; I haven't gotten a wink of sleep."

Without a good night's sleep, neither dog nor hockey great could be in good form the next day. Of course, as a vet, I had to make the puppy better, but as a Rangers fan, I needed Wayne Gretzky to get a good night's sleep. For the sake of *all* Rangers fans, I had to cure this puppy's cough ASAP.

Liberty had the classic signs of tracheobronchitis, an infectious respiratory disease commonly called kennel cough. I injected her with antibiotics and dispensed doggie cough suppressants for overnight.

"She should feel better in no time," I said.

The *second* I got outside, I called Steve. "Honey, I just met The Great One!"

"What do you mean, 'The Great One'? Like, the *great*, Great One?!" he asked incredulously. "The only person known as . . . Shut up! *No!* You did not! That's it. I'm coming on your next house call."

"I can't wait to go to the game tomorrow," I said. "And I predict he'll score."

Janet confirmed that Liberty was already feeling better the next day and she had slept quietly all night. I hoped Gretzky had, too. That evening, as we cheered to the point of hoarseness from our seats in Madison Square Garden, the great Wayne Gretzky scored a beautiful goal, and the Rangers won. But only Steve and I knew I had something to do with it.

As a house call vet, I'm sometimes exposed to sights that I'd otherwise never behold. Some have even been astonishing.

One night in the early 2000s, Steve and I were getting dressed for a performance of *The Marriage of Figaro* at the Metropolitan Opera. Our home phone rang. Steve was putting on his cuff links and he shot me a "I hope that's not a client" look. Well, if you are married to a vet, emergency cases are part of the package.

"This is Cher," said a woman over a crackly phone line. She sounded a lot like the one-named icon. "Joan Rivers gave me your home number."

I dropped my eyeliner and started pacing the bathroom with a rush of adrenaline. Steve noticed my excitement and mouthed, *Who?*

I mouthed, *Cher!*

He whispered, "Chair?"

I shook my head. The icon was still talking.

"I'm on a plane—on my way back from Italy with my new dog, Pippo. I found him on the street while filming in Rome, and I'm bringing him home with me now. He can't stop scratching himself. Joan said you make house calls."

She continued, "My plane lands at Kennedy Airport at 11:30 p.m. and then I'm going straight to the Waldorf. Can you come to the hotel at midnight?"

"You're calling from *a plane?*" I asked, amazed. *Could you actually do that?*

While I do try to accommodate my most demanding clients, I don't make house calls at midnight. However, this was Cher! I told her that I could meet her but at the animal hospital, where the overnight technician would help me with my new patient.

"I have a limo," she said. "Where do I need to go?"

I gave her the address of the hospital, and we agreed to meet there with Pippo at midnight.

Steve said, "Big night!"

"Yep, first Renée Fleming at the Met, and then Cher's Italian rescue dog at midnight. Just a typical night in the life of a Manhattan house call vet." (Early that day, I drained a pus-filled abscess from a basset hound's leg. *That* was more my typical day.)

At the end of the opera, I gave Steve a quick kiss and rushed from my seat while the rest of the audience was still in its standing ovation. Since I was one of the first to leave, I had no trouble hailing a taxi. I arrived at the hospital on time and found the limo driver in full livery already in the waiting room. He was holding a small terrier mix.

He asked, "Are you Dr. Amy? This is Pippo."

No Cher? *She sent her driver?* I had to take a second to shake off my crushing disappointment, and then focused on the dog. "Come on back to the exam room and I'll take care of Pippo," I told him.

I put a lab coat over my fancy dress, gloved up, and gave Pippo a thorough exam. He seemed healthy except for an angry, itchy rash. I had a pretty good idea from the location of the splotches what it was—a nuisance parasite called sarcoptic mange—but wanted to do some diagnostics to confirm it. I took samples from his skin and looked at them under the microscope. I immediately saw the microscopic, monster-scary parasites that were living in his skin and causing the problem.

"What Pippo has is contagious, even to people," I said to the limo driver. "I'm going to give you gloves to wear and some to take back to the hotel. Cher doesn't want to catch this. Please tell her not to share her bed or any towels with this lucky guy for a while."

He just blinked.

The treatment for sarcoptic mange at that time was an injection of ivermectin (a medication that became controversial as a Covid-19 treatment). Based on the reaction of my patients, I knew the injection really stings.

"Try to stay calm and still, Pippo," I said, preparing the needle. To the driver, I added, "Don't be alarmed if he complains."

But Pippo was a good boy. He didn't flinch when I gave him the injection. He even licked my gloved hand. "He's going to need a follow-up visit in two weeks," I told the driver. "Either here in New York or . . . wherever Cher is then."

"Thank you," he said. "I'll let Ms. Cher know. She asked me to take you anywhere you need to go when we were done."

That bit of kindness was much appreciated. It was one a.m., my feet (still in heels) were killing me, and I couldn't wait to get out of my dress and into pajamas. I was ushered to the longest stretch limousine I'd ever seen and climbed into the back. The bench seat was as long as my living room couch, and I busied myself by opening every cabinet, checking out the full bar with its crystal glassware. I wasn't interested in a drink, but I appreciated the possibilities.

When we pulled up at my building, I hoped one of my neighbors would be around to see me step out of that beast. Sadly, none were . . . but I did get a double take from our night doorman.

A few days later, Cher's assistant called me to report that Pippo was much improved.

"Cher's very happy," she said.

I smiled. "Pippo will need another injection in just over a week. How would you like to handle it?"

"Cher will still be in New York then," she said, so we arranged a time when I could come to the Waldorf-Astoria to administer the second injection.

I told Shari about the appointment. "Do you think we'll meet her?" she asked.

"I doubt it; staff probably, but at least we'll get to see a VIP suite at the Waldorf."

When I arrived at the appointed time, I was escorted by a bell-man to a floor accessible only with a special key. After a gentle knock, a young woman opened the door to a rambling, sun-drenched suite that was as stunning as I'd hoped.

"Make yourself comfortable," she instructed. "I'm Colette. I'll be right back with the dog." A quick glance around but again no sign of Cher. *Oh well.*

She carried Pippo out without gloves on and handed him to me for his exam. His rashes were greatly improved, but he still needed another injection of ivermectin.

"Be a good boy, like the other night," I urged him.

I dabbed the site with alcohol and then gently plunged the needle into his thigh.

This time when I injected the medicine, Pippo screamed bloody murder.

Into the room flew Cher herself, her dark eyes flashing fury *at me.* "What the *hell* did you do to my dog?!" she yelled.

Shari shot me a look that said, *You're in trouble now, Attas.*

I was speechless for a second as I took her in. Cher wore a hotel bathrobe, her head was full of giant hot rollers, and her face was smeared with gloppy white cream.

"Pippo is perfectly fine," I said. "The injection just stung a little."

"*Stung a little?* I could hear him from three rooms away!"

The suite had three more rooms? A tour seemed now out of the question given the circumstances.

"I didn't think he'd complain because he was so quiet the last time!" Less than two weeks in the lap of luxury, Pippo the Roman street dog had become a diva in his own right. "He's had his full treatment now and the mange should be gone soon. Just continue to be careful about touching him. It is still contagious to humans."

"*Contagious?!*" she asked aghast. I reasoned that the driver hadn't passed along my warning. "Well, that explains it. Does the rash on humans look like *this*?" And without warning, Cher flung her bathrobe open to reveal her iconic body in its naked entirety.

I gaped. Looked away. Looked back. Then I returned my gaze and locked my eyes directly on hers and asked, "Does it itch?"

"Nah," she replied, refastening her robe. "And come to think of it, I had the rash before I had Pippo. It's probably just a heat rash. It was hot in Rome."

"You're probably right," I agreed, not knowing what else to say.

Our business done, Shari and I left Cher's suite, and we could not stop laughing in the elevator on our way down. "I bet she does Pilates," said Shari.

"I know!" I agreed. "Makes me think I should start exercising more."

People often ask to see photos of me with my celebrity clients. Sadly, I don't have many. I meet these people in their homes, and I respect that this is their sanctuary from public life. It would be inappropriate to ask for a selfie in their private space. However, if we meet in public or at a performance, I feel I can ask. The only photo I have with Billy Joel was taken backstage at the Richard Rodgers Theatre, where he was a public person. When I went to see *Henry IV* starring my client Kevin Kline and went backstage, Steve took a wonderful photograph of me with Kevin in his Falstaff fat costume.

Not all vets feel the same way. Once, I referred Joan Rivers to see a veterinary ophthalmologist because I found something wrong with Spike's eye. A few years later, my own dog needed to see the same ophthalmologist. Hanging on the wall of the exam room was a photograph of her with her arm around Joan Rivers's shoulder. I thought, *I've known Joan for twenty-five years, and I don't have a single photo with her. This ophthalmologist meets her once, and now she has a best-bud photo hanging on her wall.* But I stick by my principles.

Steve Martin, a quintessential New Yorker, is another of my wonderful clients. I'm a fan of his films and books and love the series *Only Murders in the Building.* I recall a time I went to his apartment for an appointment and stood outside the closed front door just to listen to him playing his banjo inside. I knew that once I rang the bell, he would stop playing and my private concert would be over. Of course, I'd love to have a picture with him, but it would violate our understood professional relationship if I asked for it in his home, which was the only place I ever saw him. But this didn't mean I didn't *want* a photo with Steve Martin.

One day, his office called with an unusual request. He was filming *The Pink Panther* at the iconic movie and TV production facility Silvercup Studios in Long Island City, Queens. They asked if I could see Roger, his charming yellow Lab, who was on set with him all day.

Even though I don't typically venture outside of Manhattan to treat patients, I said yes to this. "Shari," I bubbled. "We're going to Queens!"

"This excites you?" she asked.

I explained the situation. "I've never been to a movie production set before. And Steve Martin's going to be in costume, right? Maybe I can get a photo with him." In this scenario, at his place of work where cameras were pointed at him all day, it seemed appropriate to ask for a quick pic.

The whole way out to Long Island City, I kept saying to Shari, "I can't believe I'm going to finally get a picture with Steve Martin!"

She laughed and said, "You are way too hyped about this, Attas."

I was, unapologetically so.

When we were granted entry into the lot, I bounced with excitement in the back seat. It was fun just to be on a movie set. Around us were two-dimensional renderings that looked fake, but I knew they would look like Paris in postproduction.

A production assistant brought us to Martin's trailer, one of those eighteen-wheel vehicles with corrugated metal steps to get to the door. A few trailers sat end to end in a row, and they looked identical from the outside. On the inside, Martin's looked like a lovely studio apartment with a queen-sized bed, a fancy living room area with beautiful furniture, and a fully functional kitchenette where you could cook a three-course meal. Of course, there was no need to cook as the catering trucks were right outside.

Roger was there, wagging his tail as he always did when he saw me. But Steve was nowhere in sight. Shari could see my disappointment. "He'll come by," she said.

She was probably right. Every time we had a visit with Roger at the apartment, Steve was always there to ask how his beloved dog was doing. Roger was his constant companion.

I began Roger's physical exam. I ran through my usual routine at half speed, then at quarter speed, stalling for as long as possible with the hope that the star would appear. Finally, right when I couldn't move any slower, he came into the trailer. I was ready.

He was in his Inspector Clouseau costume—the signature pencil mustache and trench coat of the bumbling French detective—and holding a cell phone to his ear. He nodded at us but kept talking to the person on the other end. From his tone and expression, I could tell he was upset about something. In all the years he'd been my client, I'd never heard him raise his voice before.

Shari gave me a clear-as-day nonverbal message that said, *Don't you dare ask him for a photo today!* I nodded in agreement; he was definitely not in the mood.

We packed up our stuff at a normal pace. Martin excused himself from the conversation and turned to me and asked, "Anything you need to tell me about Roger?"

"No, he's fine. I'll call you with lab results in a few days."

I sulked all the way to Manhattan across the Queensboro Bridge. I never got a photo, but being on set of a major film—not to mention in the trailer of the star—was a thrill and made for one of my standout days.

Another job perk: being able to wow out-of-town friends.

Two days after my very first house call with Billy Joel, Steve and I were hosting our friends Lori and Josh from California. They wanted to see *Movin' Out*, the jukebox Broadway musical conceived and created by the great choreographer Twyla Tharp, based on Billy's songs.

We got tickets to see it, and as we waited to enter the theater,

Steve said with the straight-faced delivery that only he can, "FYI, Billy's going to be here tonight."

He was just joking, but they believed him. Lori exclaimed, "Oh my God! Is he really?!"

"No, Steve just made that up," I corrected.

The show was indeed *wonderful*. Billy's music. Tharp's choreography. One of the best evenings of musical theater we'd ever seen. The audience stood and cheered straight through two encores. And then, when the curtain rose for the third one and we expected the cast would come out to take its final bows, there was Billy Joel! Alone onstage, seated at the piano. As Steve had said he'd be.

The crowd went nuts.

I turned to our friends and said with a glance to Steve, "I guess I'm not the only witch in the family."

Billy energetically played an encore of "Scenes from an Italian Restaurant." The audience could not stop cheering.

As we left the theater, flying on a Broadway high, I said to our group, "Come with me." Now Steve looked at me quizzically.

I led our friends to the stage door of the Richard Rodgers Theatre, pushed my way through the crowd to the front, and wrote a quick note on my business card. I got the attention of the security guard and said, "Please give this to Mr. Joel."

The stage door guard read my card and then looked at me. I explained, "I'm his veterinarian."

He replied, "I've never heard that one before." The guard went inside and came right back out and said, "Mr. Joel says you can come in."

The four of us went backstage to where Billy was hanging out with actor Paul Reiser. We all chatted for about fifteen minutes, got a great group photo, and then it was time to leave. We walked outside together, they got into their limo, and we walked to Orso and enjoyed a fabulous dinner. I'd only been working with Billy for a short time at that point, so his graciousness and the alignment of the stars (literally) enabled this incredible experience.

The fun of being Billy Joel's vet kept on coming. On a subsequent house call, Billy was staying at the Four Seasons, a luxury hotel on East 57th Street. While I was working with one of his pugs, I overheard him say, "After this, I'm going to Steinway."

Steinway Hall, the showroom for the storied piano company, Steinway & Sons, was then just a few blocks away on West 57th Street, next door to the Buckingham Hotel, where I lived.

I said, "You know, I'm right next door to Steinway, in the building where Paderewski lived and died."

The Buckingham was the final home of Ignacy Jan Paderewski, one of the greatest concert pianists and composers of his time, who was also the first prime minister of free Poland. He was loaded with personality and had a trademark head of wild, crazy hair. Mothers of that time warned their children to brush their hair or they'd "look like Paderewski." He made his American debut in 1891 at the brand-new Carnegie Hall, which is just across the street from the Buckingham and Steinway. He was the Mick Jagger of his day, who'd toured all over Europe and sold out at the old Madison Square Garden every night.

How do I know all this? Steve installed a plaque commemorating Paderewski on the front of the Buckingham. When Paderewski died in 1941, lines of his fans wanting to pay respects went for blocks down Sixth Avenue.

Billy replied, "Wow! I play one of Paderewski's pianos."

Of course he did. He probably owned one of Beethoven's, too.

"Walk with me to Steinway Hall and I'll play some of his music for you," he said.

We walked the few blocks to Steinway together, where Billy played beautiful music for a private audience of me and some of the luckiest piano shoppers who happened to be there at the moment. Not a bad day to be a New Yorker on 57th Street. Or Billy Joel's vet.

CHAPTER 11

Sex and Pets and the City

Books have always been important to me, with *All Creatures Great and Small* topping the list. Another book that had a huge impact on me was *Fear of Flying,* one of the first novels about the female sexual revolution, when I was a sixteen-year-old freshman at Barnard College. It was written by Erica Jong, also an alumna of Barnard.

Some twenty years later, the revolution continued, and I hung on every word. At that time, Candace Bushnell wrote a frank column in *The New York Observer,* the salmon-colored weekly, about her experiences in the dating world in Manhattan. Her 1996 book, *Sex and the City,* based on the columns, could be found in nearly every apartment I visited as a house call vet.

I was Candace's veterinarian while at Park East in the late 1980s, years before her book was published. And then I became Erica's vet as well. Both of these authors and books came together for me, as things often do in New York.

Candace's paper, *The New York Observer,* was owned by Arthur

Carter, a banker, professor, legendary journalist, artist, and one of City Pets' best clients. Not only did he help me get a better table at Le Cirque that night, he referred a lot of clients to me, though cautioning that he wouldn't refer *everyone* because he didn't want me so busy that he couldn't get an appointment whenever he wanted one.

One friend he *did* refer was a woman with a fifteen-year-old bichon frise who needed at-home care. My new patient, Poochini, had a heart condition and chronic UTIs. And her owner was Erica Jong.

I was excited to meet the feminist icon whose writing altered the world view of many twentieth-century women. I was also excited to see her apartment, assuming it'd be sensual and lavish, with draped fabrics and tasseled pillows on Persian rugs like a harem room or the inside of a genie's bottle. Surely, Erica would have a Sexy Life. I mean, she lived on 69th Street! In my mind, this house call could be like an episode of *Sex and the City*, the column-to-book-to-HBO-show that was a massive hit. Could I maybe play the role of Sexy Vet?

Erica's off-the-avenue building was large by Manhattan standards, with over three hundred apartments. Carida and I rode the elevator to the twenty-seventh floor with the uniformed attendant whose only job was to push the buttons.

Her apartment lived up to my imagination. Everywhere you looked, there were images of crotches and breasts with boing-y nipples. On the entry wall was a life-sized brightly colorfed neon outline of a reclining female nude by the artist Tom Wesselmann. I've glimpsed Van Goghs, a Jackson Pollock, Damien Hirsts, and other important works up close. But Erica's was my first exposure to erotic pop art.

Sadly my sexy house call turned out to be anything but. Poochini was not well. His various illnesses were a challenge to manage because treatment for one condition, kidney failure, exacerbated his other condition, heart failure. He also had another bladder infection and severe arthritis, which made walking very difficult.

I returned to Erica's erotic haven many times to fine-tune Poochini's treatments until it was time for her to let him go. She held his paw while I put Poochini, then seventeen, to sleep. Her cats, Latte and Espresso, watched nearby.

I never got my sexy house call.

Spike Rivers, Joan's Yorkie, was an extremely sexy dog. Despite being neutered, he had a girlfriend named Carmelita. Carmelita was a pink fluffy slipper that Joan had wanted to discard but couldn't because Spike made love to it often.

Regularly, I'd get a call from her house manager Kevin, "He's done it again, and it won't go back in."

"I'll be right there."

"It" was Spike's penis.

I'd find Spike in the den, spent, next to an exhausted fluffy Carmelita, his little red lipstick of a penis stuck out for all the world to see. Ordinarily, an amorous dog's penis retracts back into the external sheath, called the prepuce, after sexual activity. But Spike would go at it for so long with his furry slipper girlfriend that his penis would get too dry to slide back inside the prepuce and remain stuck outside.

Spike was so serious about his love for Carmelita that this happened frequently. The problem did not require professional veterinary care, but Joan insisted that I come over and apply the KY jelly needed to make his little manhood slippery enough so it went back in where it belonged.

Repeatedly, I showed her what I was doing and explained that she could do this for him herself.

"I'm *not* doing *that!*" she said. "No free hand jobs. Not even for Spike."

Some of my patients were more like the sex police watching over their owners.

On a recent visit to Mary and Mitch Lander, a newly married couple in their thirties, Mary shared with me, "Every time we have sex, Tyson goes crazy barking and jumping around on the bed. It's very distracting."

Tyson was a four-year-old Chihuahua who belonged to Mary from before the couple were married. They lived in a one-bedroom apartment on East 34th Street near NYU Langone hospital, where Mitch was a surgical resident. He worked long and unpredictable hours, including many overnight shifts. Since they were having difficulty getting pregnant, their sex life was scheduled around the times Mary was ovulating.

Scheduling a quickie during a lunch break was stressful enough, but lately they were unable to complete their main mission. Every time they became amorous, Tyson would bark, growl, and snap at Mitch's feet. When he eventually bit through Mitch's skin one afternoon, the little dog had crossed the line and prevented Mitch and Mary from crossing their goal line.

They called me wanting to know why Tyson was such an annoying little sex blocker.

"Tell me about your relationship with Tyson," I asked Mary.

"We're together 24/7. Whenever I go out, I take him with me in

200

my purse like Paris Hilton does," she told me, smiling adoringly at Tyson.

"A dog who is so bonded with someone can become highly protective," I explained. "When your husband is doing something that looks like he might be hurting you, Tyson is trying to stop it. I explained that the sounds and activities that they were engaged in probably looked to Tyson like they were in a fight.

"What can we do about it? We tried locking him in the bathroom, but he went crazy and scratched the door until his nails bled," she said.

"He can still hear you from the bathroom," I explained. "He was probably frantic because he couldn't protect you. Tyson must leave the apartment when you have sex."

Mary looked at me like I was crazy. "Where would he go?"

I thought for a moment and then asked, "Do you have a neighbor who can take Tyson during your lunchtime appointments?"

She smiled. "We do. My next-door neighbor is a freelance writer who loves Tyson. She's home all day, and I bet she'd take him for an hour." Then she added, "Though with my husband's schedule it might be more like fifteen minutes!" And we both laughed.

And that was how they worked it out. The neighbor babysat Tyson while the couple got busy. They eventually had twins. Tyson wasn't happy about those newcomers, either.

Back in my Park East days, I met Diva, a large female briard, who belonged to Alison and Bill. The couple were in their early sixties, semi-retired, and enjoyed their time off by taking Diva to field dog trials. They traveled weekends bringing her to events, and she had become quite accomplished.

They called early one day, concerned about Diva. She didn't eat her dinner the night before, which was very unusual for her. They reported that she'd vomited all night, and this morning was repeatedly attempting to vomit, but nothing was coming out. I told them to come right to the hospital.

Animals can't describe their problems, so I have to rely both on my observations and what the owners tell me. I'm an animal medicine detective. In the course of my inquiry, Alison said that Diva had been known to eat things she wasn't supposed to.

As I examined Diva, I made my own findings. Her belly was painful when I palpated it, and there was a piece of elastic fabric wrapped around her tongue that extended down her throat into her esophagus, the food pipe.

"Diva has eaten something she shouldn't have," I reported.

"But she hasn't eaten any food in over a day," reported Alison.

"I don't think it's food. I'll need to X-ray her to better understand what's going on."

The X-ray showed Diva's stomach was completely full and also that her intestines were bunched together. The elastic under her tongue was attached to whatever she'd swallowed and was filling her stomach. Her intestines were desperately trying to move the foreign material along but couldn't because the material was anchored around her tongue.

Most of my vomiting patients get treated with fluids and medications, but Diva needed immediate surgery to remove the foreign material. The appearance of bunched intestines on the X-ray could mean that the intestinal blood supply was compromised. If this wasn't remedied quickly, it could be fatal.

As soon as Diva was under anesthesia, I cut the elastic under her tongue so the tugging on her intestines would stop. After cutting into her abdomen, I focused my attention on her stomach and intestines. I made my first incision into her stomach where I saw the offending item. It was a woman's silk half-slip, the bulk of which was in Diva's stomach. I removed as much as I could, but a portion was still stuck in her intestine. I made two small incisions into the angry red gut and removed the remaining silk material. Diva had eaten the entire undergarment and might have actually passed it on her own if the elastic waist band hadn't gotten caught under her tongue. In the time it took to suture the incisions closed, the intestines were contracting and returning to their normal pink color, indicating that the blood supply was still intact.

When the surgery was over and Diva was in recovery, I put the soggy, smelly slip into a Ziploc bag and brought it out to the waiting room where Diva's family was waiting and showed it to them.

"So that's where my slip went," Alison remarked, shaking her head. "I looked everywhere for it."

Diva's case was unusual because she kept eating ladies' undergarments. I removed from her stomach some very sheer gray stockings, a pair of sexy midnight-blue silk panties, and an elaborately harem-style decorated underwire bra whose outline was distinctive on the X-ray. I'm not sure this was a case of Diva eating everything lying around; rather, I suspect Diva (and her mom, too?) had a lingerie fetish.

Meanwhile, Diva was so popular that she always had a large audience when she was in weekend show events. At one event, Diva stopped in the middle of the field and vomited up a black thong bikini. In front of everybody.

At first glance, Alison glared at her husband and shrieked loudly, *"Those aren't mine!"*

He had a look of terror on his face but in a few moments they both laughed when they remembered that Diva dove under the hotel bed when they arrived the night before and came out swallowing something. Apparently she ate somebody else's thong.

Although this didn't present any marital issues, the incident did raise concerns about the quality of their hotel's housekeeping. They resolved not to stay there again.

It's generally agreed that it's hard to get dogs to take a pill even when it's wrapped up in a delicious morsel of food. They greedily gobble up the meat or cheese and then cleverly spit out the pill when you're not looking. They are darn good at it, particularly when they give you that "Nope, nothing to see here" look afterward. In fact, dogs are so notorious for this behavior that pet food companies make special "fool 'em" products to try to help get the pills down, like a tasty little Tootsie Roll that you can hide a pill inside.

So why then, when it is so hard to get them to take their own meds, do dogs scarf up human medication the second we drop one of our pills on the kitchen floor?

Oscar, a nine-month-old Cavalier King Charles spaniel, wouldn't take his pills. It was a constant struggle each month to get him to swallow his heartworm prevention.

Oscar belonged to the Shaws, an elderly couple who lived on East 65th Street and Park Avenue. In every outward respect, they were proper blue bloods. Mrs. Shaw always dressed in Chanel, and Mr. Shaw wore three-piece suits with regimental ties, even on Sundays. I was surprised when they opted to get a puppy after their elderly dog passed away, since a puppy is a lot for a couple in their eighties. Though Oscar was a handful, the Shaws doted on him like a grandchild.

Mrs. Shaw, normally quiet and reserved, called one evening in hysterics. "Dr. Amy! I just caught Oscar standing on my husband's night table chewing on something. I pulled out a partially eaten vial of my husband's pills, and I think Oscar ate some of them. *I have no idea what they are because he ate the label, too.*"

"Okay, take a deep breath. Let's do a process of elimination and see if we can figure this out," I said. "Do you have a list of his prescriptions?"

She cried, "No! And I can't reach my husband. He's at the Harvard Club. I left word to call as soon as possible."

Just then her landline rang. It was Mr. Shaw. He apologized and said that he had been playing squash for the past hour. She quickly told him what happened and put both phones on speaker next to each other so the three of us could hear what everyone was saying.

"Let's run down every pill you take," I said to Mr. Shaw, "and your wife can check if they're still on the nightstand."

He said, "Okay. There's Lipitor."

"Yes, I see it," said Mrs. Shaw. "It hasn't been chewed on."

"And Eliquis and Celebrex . . ."

"Yes, I have those, too. Also unchewed. They're all here. *What's missing?!*"

I wanted to say how impressed I was that he could play an hour of squash at his age with high blood pressure, arthritis, and atrial fibrillation. Modern medicine to the rescue.

"Well, there is one more," he said, sounding a bit sheepish.

"What is it?" Mrs. Shaw and I both asked at the same time.

He said, "It's . . . it's the one for men."

Mrs. Shaw got it. "Oh my God, Oscar ate the Viagra!" she said. "Yes, that has to be it. The Viagra! The vial is chewed up and empty!"

As if that review wasn't embarrassing enough for me to be party to, the next step was to estimate *how many* Viagra pills Oscar had eaten. And to do this, we had to start from the total number prescribed and then determine how many the Shaws had used since the prescription was filled.

"Okay, the prescription was refilled three weeks ago," he said. "It started with thirty."

"So . . . how many times have we . . . um . . . in the last three weeks?" Mrs. Shaw whispered.

"Well, sweetheart, let's see. I know there was the dinner party. And then after the gala." I had a sense he forgot that I was there. Together, with me listening in to an accounting of their sex calendar over the past three weeks, the Shaws figured out that Oscar must have eaten sixteen pills. Meaning this proper, elderly couple had had sex *fourteen times in the last twenty-one days*. Now *that's* a miracle of modern science.

I paused to take that in and mentally paid them the proper respect. And then, in pure doctor mode, I said, "Oscar eating sixteen Viagra is a genuine problem."

I confirmed that with a quick call to Animal Poison Control, a twenty-four-hour service available for vets and clients. Such a large quantity of Viagra in a dog of Oscar's weight was dangerous. It might affect his heart and could cause seriously low blood pressure. He would have to be admitted to the hospital for blood pressure control and overnight observation.

"I'm already on my way to the hospital," said Mrs. Shaw.

The next day, when Oscar was cleared to go home, Mr. Shaw picked him up. I called them in the evening to find out how the dog was feeling. I'm sure Mr. Shaw smiled when he said, "What a waste of Viagra on Oscar since you neutered him two weeks ago," he joked.

He was in a good mood, and we both laughed. In the back of my mind, I couldn't help but wonder if the Shaws had already refilled the prescription and subtracted one last night.

It's widely acknowledged that the best kind of sex is spontaneous. But as a house call vet, I have to say that there are times that isn't true. George and I had been making monthly visits to treat a bulldog with chronic Lyme disease. The owner told me that no one would be home, and they would leave the door open. I would find the dog in the kitchen of their Park Avenue apartment. After we were finished with our patient, George said, "I'm going to take advantage of no one being home and find a bathroom while you clean up."

A thing about being a house call vet: We are in constant anxiety about bathroom access during our workday. Most clients never think to offer use of theirs, and sometimes it's too awkward to ask, so we wait until we park near a Starbucks, stop at the clinic, or are alone in a client's apartment.

Normally, this client was home for their dog's treatment, and we'd never been anywhere but the kitchen. So, George—in need—went in search of a powder room, walking down the central corridor, opening doors at random.

While packing up our stuff in the kitchen, I heard him yell, "Oh my God!"

Then I heard a young woman yell back, "Oh my God!"

George came running back into the kitchen, red-faced, saying, "Let's go! Let's go!"

We grabbed our stuff and ran out to the elevator. Once we were inside, he started laughing.

"What happened?" I asked, laughing along without knowing why.

"I opened a door and found two teenagers in bed," he said.

The family had a son who was supposed to be in school. I guess he thought he could play hooky for nookie with his girlfriend while his parents were both at work.

We never breathed a word of it to his parents, and neither did he. And, of course, we continued to treat the bulldog for Lyme disease, but after that always rang the doorbell even when they told us no one would be home. I wish I remembered to do that everywhere.

CHAPTER 12

I'm Beautiful, so My Pet Must Be, Too

In the wild, animals flaunt their physical characteristics in competition for mates. Think of brightly colored birds or stags showing off their huge racks, all designed to look great to attract the opposite sex. But in the concrete jungle of Manhattan, neutered pets have no biological reason to care what other cats or dogs think about how they look, nor are they aware of their appearance even if they recognize themselves in a mirror.

But animal attractiveness *does* apparently matter to their people, particularly to some of my Manhattan clients. They often seek out a particular breed simply because of how it looks. The breed's attributes are ones that *humans* declare attractive, even though they don't make a difference from the animal's point of view. The winner of the dog show doesn't feel better-looking than the runners-up.

Most of my clients love their pets unconditionally. But there have been a handful whose personal issues with vanity were an essential element of their relationship with their pet, to the point that their obsession with their pet's appearance made it hard for me to provide their animals the best medical care.

The first day I met Roberta and Richard Glassman at Park East, they were sitting in the waiting room with what I thought was a giant fawn pug nestled between them. The dog was actually an English mastiff puppy named Taft, who would grow up to be the size of a refrigerator. Roberta and Richard would both come to every one of Taft's puppy vaccine appointments, and they were ideal clients who followed all my instructions. Except for one.

When Taft turned a year old, we had a sit-down talk about getting him neutered. I'd broached the subject before, and now that it was time, I did it again. But the Glassmans told me that they weren't ready. When Taft was closer to two and fully grown, I brought it up again.

I told them all the reasons I recommended the surgery. "There are both health and personality benefits," I explained. "An un-neutered male dog might become aggressive with other animals because of his testosterone level. It can make other animals aggressive toward him, particularly a dog as big as Taft. Importantly, it also increases his risk of developing certain medical problems like prostate disease. Neutering is considered the 'standard of care' for dogs."

Roberta listened intently, but I could see that Richard had a resolute and defiant look on his face. "No dog of mine is going to have his balls cut off," he spat out the instant I finished talking. "He's a tough dog, and I don't want him to look like a girl. He was born to have them hanging, and that's what he's going to have." Richard himself was large and assertive, and I sensed that this concern was somewhat self-reflective.

I didn't have to worry about Taft being aggressive. He might have looked scary, but he was a gentle giant with a heart full of love. Even unneutered, he was the sweetest 160-pound drool machine I'd ever met.

The Glassmans were never home when we made house calls to their prewar, two-bedroom rental apartment on West End Avenue. It had great bones, but they'd made little effort to furnish or decorate it. It looked like they'd just moved in and were waiting for the furniture to arrive. The kitchen was small, and I never saw any signs of its use, but that wasn't surprising since they owned several popular Manhattan restaurants. They probably ate out every night, so why bother stocking the pantry, much less turning on the stove?

The Glassmans' doorman always smiled when I arrived at the building because I gave him free advice about his cat each time. "Who are you here to see today, Doc?" he asked.

"The big boy," I replied, and he handed me the keys to the Glassmans' apartment.

As soon as I inserted the key in the lock I heard Taft's nails on the parquet floor followed by his thunderous bark as he ran headlong toward the door and its visitor. Normally, I wouldn't enter the home of a *ginormous*, unneutered male dog when no one was home, but I did with Taft. I turned the key and slowly opened the door wide enough so he could see me. As soon as he did, he stopped dead in his tracks, sliding a few feet, and then turned 180 degrees and ran off into another room.

Many of my patients run *from* me when they see me. Not Taft. He returned, also on the run, two seconds later with a giant stuffed hedgehog in his mouth for us to play with together. He dropped the drool-saturated toy right at my feet and gave me the most hopeful, heart-squeezing look with a wag of his entire hindquarters.

211

Taft didn't mind if I gave him injections or performed other indignities. He just loved my attention, and he returned my affection. When my medical work was done, I always overstayed my allotted time for a good dose of Taft-love and play.

When Taft was six, he had medical issues. The Glassmans reported he was drinking a lot of water and urinating around the apartment. The predictable diagnoses—diabetes, a UTI, kidney disease, or liver disease—could be determined by blood and urine tests. I went to this house call prepared to get those samples.

The Glassmans were home. Taft brought me his favorite toy, but I could see that his heart wasn't in it. While doing my exam he flinched when I palpated his groin region. He cried when I lifted his tail and inserted my gloved finger into his rectum to examine his prostate gland.

Through the rectal wall, the prostate should feel like a large lychee nut: smooth, symmetrical, bilobed, and slightly compressible. But Taft's gland was enlarged and irregular, and he winced when I touched it. I couldn't make a definitive diagnosis with just a finger's examination. Further diagnostics would tell if it was a benign prostatic hypertrophy, a prostatic infection, or cancer. I just knew that my dear Taft had prostate cancer, a diagnosis that would make the remainder of his now-shortened life uncomfortable.

Richard, watching, could see the distress on my face. "How bad is it?" he asked.

"Taft has a problem with his prostate," I told the couple. "I will submit my blood and urine samples and make the arrangements to do an ultrasound-guided biopsy so I can know for sure if it is an infection or cancer. But I think it is cancer."

Roberta broke down crying and through her tears, she asked, "Is this because we didn't neuter him?"

Richard dropped his gaze to the bare floor of the living room but said nothing. I wondered if his insistence not to neuter Taft had come up between them over the years. I was sure there'd be an intense conversation after I left.

"Probably . . . yes," I answered. I didn't add anything to that. It would have been cruel to blame the dog's disease on Richard's long-ago choice, even if it was the wrong one. I could see he already had enough guilt without me piling on.

I went back to veterinarian mode. "Let's talk about next steps. After we get back the labs and the biopsy of his prostate, we can then develop a treatment protocol."

"We'll do whatever needs to be done," said Roberta and Richard in unison.

The biopsy confirmed that Taft had aggressive prostate cancer. It wasn't possible to surgically remove the tumor, so Taft started chemotherapy. He didn't respond well to the treatment even after I reduced the dosage. He was sick for days each time he received the chemo.

The Glassmans and I agreed that we should discontinue his chemo after the third round. Soon after, my big friend could no longer go on his long walks, and with merely the slightest exertion, he had difficulty breathing. His disease had metastasized into his lungs. The Glassmans knew that Taft needed to be put to sleep to end his obvious suffering, but like others often do, they held out till the very last moment.

The upcoming Valentine's Day was the five-year anniversary of my engagement with Steve. We would be celebrating that evening at Café des Artistes, one of our favorite romantic restaurants. I had arranged to finish house calls early that day to go home, wash my hair, and spend a little extra time on my makeup. I put on a new red silk dress for the occasion.

We were heading out the door when my pager vibrated. I looked down at the screen. It read, "Call Glassmans ASAP."

Roberta picked up but I couldn't understand what she was saying because of her sobs. What I finally understood was, "Taft can't breathe. We need you now."

"I'll be there as quickly as I can."

Steve called the restaurant to change our reservation while I called George to ask him to meet me at the Glassmans'.

George looked surprised when he saw me in my fancy dress and high heels. It was indeed a little awkward when we sat on the floor around Taft, my dress a little too short and tight to do this easily. Once in position, Roberta cradled Taft's huge head and Richard held one of his paws.

I picked up Taft's other front leg and inserted a butterfly catheter, through which I injected the cocktail of medications that would first sedate him and then painlessly stop his heart.

As I worked, tears streamed from my eyes and my carefully applied makeup ran down my face and onto my new red dress. Taft passed peacefully, and when it was appropriate, I gathered my things and quietly left after giving them both a hug. George stayed behind to wait for the emergency crematorium service to pick up Taft's body.

Back home, Steve answered the door ready to go out for our dinner. He took one look at me and said, "Let's just stay in." He handed me a drink and we ate leftovers.

Ten months later, it was New Year's Eve, and Steve and I were at our weekend home for the holiday. It was a beautiful evening, almost as bright as daytime with the full moon reflecting off the crystals of the snow. We were heading out to a party when my pager went off at nine p.m.

I dialed my answering service and was told that Richard Glassman called with an emergency. *Richard?* I couldn't imagine what the emergency could be. To the best of my knowledge, he didn't even have a dog.

Once again, with one foot out the door heading to a celebration, I returned his call. "Hello, Richard. What's going on? What's the emergency?"

"We think we've identified a new puppy and I just want to talk to you about him."

That's the emergency? "I'm glad to hear that, Richard. But nine o'clock on New Year's Eve is not a good time. Can we talk about this during business hours?" I put him off with respect, which he hadn't shown me by calling when he did and labeling it an emergency.

Three weeks later, Richard and Roberta brought home Wilson, a magnificent male English mastiff puppy with dark brown fur and soulful eyes. Wilson was another great dog, and he clearly brought joy to the Glassmans. They celebrated Wilson's one-year birthday with a party at one of their restaurants with all their friends and me in attendance.

After his birthday, I began my campaign to strongly urge them to neuter Wilson. I didn't say, "If you do it, he won't die a painful, traumatizing death like Taft did," but I did hope that my unspoken message was received.

Roberta was all for it. "Of course we will."

But once again, Richard was adamant. "No, we won't."

Now I had to be explicit. "Neutering him could prevent him from getting prostate cancer," I said.

"No," he said. "My dog is going to look like he was born to look."

I stared at Richard, trying to discern through his eyes the motivation for this obstinance. To me it appeared to be about him and his ego. Richard was a large, dominant man, and his dog was going to have impressive testicles to affirm both his and Richard's status as alpha males. It seemed absurd to me and, I thought, to Roberta as well. I left that day with a no but made sure they knew the decision was against my medical advice.

Whenever I saw Roberta, I reminded her, "It's not too late to neuter him." My job was to do the best medicine possible for Wilson, so I persisted.

At one of those visits, she replied, "Dr. Amy, I want to, really, but I can't. Even if we did it when Richard is out of town, he would know as soon as he looked at Wilson. He's all about those balls."

"Roberta, you just gave me an idea. There is this product that I've read about called Neuticles. They're scrotal implants. Falsies. We can neuter Wilson and implant them solely for appearance. Wilson will look the same, but he won't have the testosterone the testicles produce, and that will reduce his chances of getting prostate disease."

I regretted telling her as soon as the words were out, since I couldn't perform this surgery against the wishes of the owner. But then, as if reading my mind, Roberta said, "You know, Wilson is technically *my* dog. *I* found him, paid for him, and signed the contract with the breeder." She took a breath. "I authorize you to neuter him and implant the fake balls."

The next time Richard was out of town, that was exactly what we did. Wilson was neutered and the silicon prosthetics were inserted into his scrotum. By the time Richard returned from his trip, Wilson was fully recovered. He ran to Richard to greet him with his large, very visible testicles swinging as if nothing had ever happened. Wilson and Richard slobbered over each other as they always did, and Richard didn't sense anything was amiss.

He never mentioned to me that he knew anything about it. And I surely didn't ask Roberta if she ever told him.

This was a difficult decision for me because I believe in clear communication and transparency. But in Wilson's case, the ends justified the means. And Roberta, his rightful owner, wanted to do everything possible to keep him healthy with the memory of Taft's illness still in the forefront of her mind. Richard's objection seemed to be about his own ego and his sense of his dog's manly appearance, and likely his own. But since I hadn't altered any of that, it seemed like a win-win.

Marina Romanoff, model-gorgeous though not an actual model, lived on Fifth Avenue. She had a lustrous mane of all shades of brown hair that curled perfectly at the ends and probably required monthly visits to the colorist. Her face was pale and innocent with dark brown eyes, and she had a figure that was both curvy and slim at the same time. She was always impeccably dressed in tan and brown colors that highlighted her beautiful hair. Her charming Russian accent was liltingly European, like she'd left Moscow as a young girl to study at the Sorbonne before landing in New York, though I didn't know any details of her journey.

Marina had four regal Pekingese dogs. They had cute little faces and large, dark brown eyes above their upturned noses. Each dog had long fur in all shades of brown that was groomed to a high sheen. If she'd chosen a dog breed based solely on its compatibility with her own gorgeous looks, she'd nailed it.

Her building in the East 60s had a heavy gothic décor. The doorman directed me and George through a marble arch to the elevator, which took us up to her eleventh-floor three-bedroom. The doors opened directly into her grand apartment, and the four dogs rushed over in their rolling gaits with long-haired tails wagging. At first glance, they looked like pushmi-pullyus, the fictional animal from the Doctor Doolittle books whose back end you couldn't tell from its front.

At that first visit, it took me a second to get over the shock of Marina's beauty and her similarly coiffed, beautiful Pekes. She led us through an apartment that was as immaculate and elegant as she was, with Central Park views out of every window. With this pack of long-haired dogs, you'd expect to see some fur on the carpet and furniture or fur balls floating in the corners of the parquet floors. Not here. There must have been a crew of housekeepers who trailed the dogs all day long and removed every trace of their hair. But oddly, I never saw anyone other than Marina in this massive apartment.

She was at home, alone, on a Thursday afternoon, decked out in Chanel. *Where does all the money come from? Does she own this place? Does she have a job, or was she born rich? Is there a wealthy partner or benefactor of some kind?* I tried not to make any assumptions and just focused on her dogs.

Marina had called us about Vlad, her five-year-old. "Something is wrong with him," she said with that charming accent. "He stays at his food bowl for a very long time, but I am not certain he is eating that much."

As part of my exam, I looked inside Vlad's mouth.

Whoa! His breath could peel the paint off the ceiling. He cried when I touched his jaw.

"Marina, Vlad has a problem in his mouth. I can't tell how serious it is without an X-ray," I explained.

She offered to take him right to the hospital for the imaging.

"It's more complicated than that," I said. "He needs to have general anesthesia to have X-rays of both his teeth and their roots. We will scale away years of tartar accumulation to see what his teeth look like. He's got a lot of bacteria in his mouth that's inflaming his gums and probably causing an infection in the tooth roots. The horrible smell is probably an infection."

Her brown eyes got very wide, and she started waving me—and the recommendation—away so hard that her Bulgari bangles clanged against each other. "He will *not* go under general anesthesia. I'll do anything you say for his teeth, but not that. No. I will use toothpaste, toothbrush."

"Brushing won't cure an infection or rotting teeth. And I need the X-ray to know the full extent of this problem."

"He will be put under, and he will never wake up," she said, her voice going up a few octaves. "I can't do that. There must be some other way."

Marina outright refused the plan, so the best I could offer was an antibiotic injection and a lesson on oral hygiene. I felt obliged to enter into Vlad's record that the client had rejected my medical plan.

Back in the elevator going down to the lobby, George turned to me and suggested, "Russian oligarch's daughter, ex-wife, or girlfriend?" He was always speculating on things like this and, in fact, had a surprising reservoir of juicy information about up-scale Manhattanites at his fingertips.

A month later she reported that Vlad was worse. "He smells very bad, and he looks swollen."

This time when I looked in Vlad's mouth, I didn't need an X-ray to see how serious it was. The swelling was hard, and it emanated from his jaw in the same place where he was painful a month before.

"This is more than an infection. Vlad may have a tumor," I said. It was impossible to know if the chronic inflammation in his mouth was part of the secret sauce that allows a tumor to grow, or if Vlad was biologically programmed to get cancer (or both). Regardless, he needed immediate intervention. "If the diagnosis is confirmed," I said, "he will have to have surgery."

"No surgery! No anesthesia!" she insisted.

I had to wonder where her anxiety over anesthesia came from. Did she know someone who died on the table? "If this is cancer and he doesn't have surgery, this will get bigger and worse. And it is truly hurting him."

Marina consented to X-rays since the first round could be done with just sedation. His chest X-ray showed no evidence of disease, but his jaw X-ray was compatible with a severe infection or jaw cancer.

I returned to discuss the imaging with Marina and did not sugarcoat the news. "He *must* go under anesthesia to have the bump biopsied and cultured. I need to know what it is in order to recommend the best way to treat it."

She consented to the biopsy, which unfortunately confirmed that Vlad had cancer in his jaw. The only treatment option was to surgically remove half of his mandible, the lower part of the jaw.

Marina looked absolutely horrified when I told her this. "No, I cannot allow this," she said. "He will look so ugly with no jaw."

Up until now, her objection was fear of anesthesia. And now, her objection to the life-saving surgery was Vlad's *appearance*? Did she think if Vlad was missing part of his jaw, he'd no longer fit into the otherwise perfect, beautiful world she had created?

"Well," I explained, "it is true that if a person had this surgery, it would be disfiguring. But it's different for a dog. He doesn't know the concept of disfigurement, so there's no psychological impact on him. And his dog friends don't care, either. In any case, his long fur would help cover it."

"His tongue will hang out of his mouth?" she asked, now finding another appearance-based objection.

"Possibly." The teeth in that region would be removed along with the jawbone, so Vlad's tongue would probably hang out. Despite that, he would be able to eat and drink just fine, albeit a bit messily.

"No. No. Vlad is too beautiful," she said. "He will never be beautiful again."

I changed my approach. Her opposition wasn't about the impact on Vlad's psyche or ego. It was about her own and her sense of the role personal beauty played in her life.

"Marina, tell me, is he beautiful now with that awful cancerous bump and with a face that tells you he is in such pain?"

I'd expected her to relent and say, "Oh my God, of course, do whatever you can to make my dog better."

But what she expressed instead was simple. "I cannot have an ugly dog," she replied without a trace of awareness of what this would mean for Vlad.

I had to wonder, *Is she just heartless or pathologically superficial?* Eventually, however, the thought of her dog Vlad not eating and living in unbearable pain cut through both her fear of general anesthesia and her peculiar fixation on her dog's beauty. Marina finally relented and agreed to the surgery.

I confess this is a ghastly procedure. The front quarter of Vlad's right jaw from the midline halfway toward the back had to be removed. While he was anesthetized, Vlad's remaining teeth were cleaned, and a full dozen completely rotten, infected stumps were extracted.

Marina didn't want to see him for the first five days after surgery. He was on intravenous narcotic therapy for the pain and being a little out of it, he drooled blood-tinged saliva. On day six, he was sufficiently improved that he no longer needed pain medication, and he began licking a soupy mixture of food from a bowl. A lot of it sprayed the walls of his kennel as he lapped, and I was pretty sure that was going to be a problem in Marina's immaculate home.

But Vlad lived on. And for the rest of his life, his tongue hung out the side of his mouth, perhaps making him slightly less regal-looking, although I thought it added to his charm. His face was much fuller on the left side than on the right where half his jaw was missing, though his long fur did much to conceal the asymmetry. But he was alive and pain free. I feared that Marina would love him less, but in the end, I never saw any change in her feeling toward him.

I'm not a psychologist, but I wonder if Marina, a woman who cared so much about her own attractiveness and that of everything surrounding her, had worried she herself would be somehow diminished if her dogs were no longer lovely. We certainly never discussed it, but I hope that loving Vlad so deeply despite his deformity helped her learn that her own value came not from her appearance, as beautiful as it was, but from her good heart, the one that made the decision to let Vlad live despite what his appearance meant for her.

Another client who was obsessed with her pets' appearance was a woman known around the world for being obsessed with her own. Joan Rivers had plastic surgery every August. She went in, got "tightened and pruned," and came out feeling refreshed. I mean, she even wrote a book about her love of plastic surgery called *Men*

Are Stupid . . . and They Like Big Boobs: A Woman's Guide to Beauty through Plastic Surgery.

Joan was one of my most loyal clients even before I started my house call practice. She recommended me freely and had me care for the procession of dogs that passed through her life. And we were friends.

First, it was Spike the Yorkie.

Next, it was Veronica, another Yorkie, whom she adopted to keep Spike company.

Then Samantha, a Havanese, followed by Max, a Pekingese.

In the mid-2000s, Joan got engaged to banker Orin Lehman, the great-grandson of Mayer Lehman who, with his brothers, founded the Lehman Brothers investment bank. Orin gave Joan a Boston terrier puppy, Lulu, for their engagement. I went to examine Lulu and wished Joan the best on her engagement.

"Congratulations! When are you getting married?" I asked.

She looked at me like I'd gone mad. *"Married?* Who said I'm getting married? I'm just getting engaged." The couple never did tie the knot. That was Joan. She had a very particular view of life.

Everything about Lulu was remarkable. She was the biggest Boston terrier I'd ever met. Ordinarily, they maxed out at fifteen pounds, but Lulu was nearly double that, tipping the doggie scale at twenty-nine pounds on a skinny day. She didn't exactly fit into Joan's eight-pound lapdog, travel-everywhere lifestyle, but Lulu was just the sweetest creature, with intelligent pointy ears and almost human eyes. A major bonus, Lulu was always formally dressed in a tuxedo, courtesy of the pattern of her own fur.

Joan loved her. We all did. Lulu was a total character.

One day out with her dog walker, this twenty-nine-pound short-legged beast leaped six feet straight up in the air and caught a pigeon in her mouth! It would be amazing if an Irish setter did that. But a Boston terrier? It was the stuff of legend.

Once, I was walking through Central Park and Lulu saw me. She *dragged* her dog walker over to get to me.

The dog walker, a woman I hadn't met yet, said, "I'm so sorry, she's never done this to anybody before."

"It's okay," I said. "She loves me." I bent down to pat her head, and she drenched my face with kisses. Most of my patients don't kiss me, but Lulu was exuberant in her affection.

When Lulu was ten, she fell off the couch and started limping. The injury was to her right hind leg. Typically, limping dogs get rest and pain medication, and a few days later, the limp is gone. But this wasn't the case with Lulu. Despite rest, she continued limping and showed no improvement after a full week.

I sent Lulu to a veterinary orthopedist for X-rays.

"Lulu has arthritis and some age-related issues," he told me. "But I see something abnormal on her right leg. I want to biopsy it."

Based on the location and its appearance on the X-rays, the orthopedist wanted to rule out osteosarcoma, an aggressive, painful bone cancer. With Lulu under anesthesia, the surgeon removed a small core of the affected bone. The results took a week to come back and confirmed the problem was osteosarcoma.

Years before, Joan courageously had me explain Spike's biopsy results live on-air during her radio show. It turned out that this encouraged listeners to bring their pets to their own vets after they checked and found lumps on them. She essentially did a public service announcement and undoubtedly saved many lives by doing it.

This time, I was relieved that Joan no longer had a radio show. The lab results were the worst diagnosis I'd ever given her.

I went to Joan's apartment on East 62nd Street and Fifth

Avenue to give her the results in person. The apartment was renowned, often written about in architecture and design magazines, a three-story mini-Versailles with wall frescos, crystal chandeliers, velvet settees, silver tea services, and all the comforts of a small palace. In that setting, I told her about Lulu's cancer and what it meant for her.

"Why didn't you just remove the damn tumor when you biopsied it?" she asked, testily.

"Well, at the time of that biopsy surgery, we didn't know what it was. And now that we do know, we also know that there is no way to remove just the tumor with this cancer. The tumor is affecting more bone than we can see. And likely it will spread." I paused. Joan's eyes drilled into mine, waiting.

"The only option is amputation," I said.

She didn't hesitate for a second. "That's not going to happen. No, I'm never going to let you remove my dog's leg. I can't look at her like that."

"She has cancer. She's in real pain. It will spread. I don't see that you have a choice. When her leg is gone, she will have no more pain."

"No, no, no, and no."

I wasn't that surprised to hear her initial objection. I knew that Joan told jokes about unattractive, overweight, and even disabled people in her stand-up act, which I assumed was just Joan pushing comedic boundaries. But here she was objecting to how Lulu's amputation would *look*, despite its benefit. But thinking about it, I mean, Joan was a beauty perfectionist. All this made understandable the thought of her beautiful Lulu becoming an amputee more than she could bear.

Joan had never before said no to any treatment I recommended for any of her dogs. Spike had lived to be sixteen and a half, a very long life for a dog, and he had a multitude of ailments including heart disease and kidney disease at the end of his life. There were weekly house calls to Veronica to express her perpetually impacted anal glands. Joan had always given me carte blanche to do everything I thought necessary. But not this time.

"I'm just not doing it. She wouldn't be Lulu anymore."

"She'll be the same funny dog—in fact, *better,* because her pain will be gone."

"I can't look at her Frankenstein scar every day!" she insisted.

I took a breath and replied bluntly, "Then we need to talk about when and where we're going to put Lulu to sleep."

Joan said, "Don't tell me what to do, Amy."

I would never! I'd learned not to question her wishes early on in our vet-client relationship. She was usually gracious about my advice, whether she followed it or not, but she had her limits. Our first real conflict happened when she brought Spike into Park East the tenth time for the same stomach trouble. "It seems to happen whenever we come home from a trip," she told me as I administered the usual fluids. "I don't think Spike really enjoys flying."

"Of course he doesn't!" I said back then, sounding more exasperated than I meant to. "Only a superdog could handle a schedule like yours. Spike is getting older, and he is having a hard time keeping up with you. It's debilitating for small animals to take long coast-to-coast flights like you do." We *all* get dehydrated on airplanes, but it happens to small dogs much more quickly, and that can be dangerous for them.

Joan's eyes got wide and her head dollied back on her graceful neck like a python getting ready to strike. "I didn't ask you how I should care for my own animal," she hissed. "I only ask you to make him better."

Oops, too far, I thought. "Okay, understood," I murmured. I got a crystal-clear understanding of the rules of our relationship: Do not question the judgment of Joan. I carried that lesson with me.

But with Lulu, I had to be resolute. This was cancer, and she was in pain.

Looking for support, I gathered the other people who loved Lulu. Joan's staff—her housekeeper, assistants, house sitters, dog walkers, dog sitters—all came together to discuss what was going on. When I told the group that Lulu had a painful bone cancer, everyone started crying. They knew and loved Joan and understood that it would be hard if not impossible for her to look at a three-legged Lulu.

A day later, Kevin and Debbie, the married couple who ran Joan's household, called me. Kevin said, "We've got an idea."

"Tell me." I was desperate for a solution.

"Would it be possible to hide the area of the amputation from Joan so that she didn't have to see it? If she doesn't see it, it'll be much easier for her."

This wasn't just a good idea; it was a *great* idea.

I knew that Lulu would feel so much better following the amputation. It's amazing how ambulatory dogs are with just three legs, especially if the affected limb is a back leg. Front-leg amputations are harder because a dog's head is heavy, and they have to hold it up while balancing on just one front foot.

So how to hide the rear incision site, which we all thought was Joan's biggest objection? With fashion, of course! Kevin, Debbie, and I designed and created tutus for Lulu, little skirts with an elastic waistband so they would stay on her tubular body. We took several dog factors into consideration, like a hem length that would accommodate Lulu when she squatted to urinate. We made the skirts longer over her back and shorter underneath so she could run and walk freely, while making sure there was enough tulle to cover the surgical site from Joan's gaze.

And the disguise worked. Joan was tickled by the wardrobe and never again mentioned the surgical site, much less Lulu's missing leg. And newly three-legged Lulu was now both pain-free and fashionable.

Ultimately, the innately good person of Joan Rivers had overcome the persona of Joan Rivers.

Lulu had no problem with losing a leg, nor did she mind wearing her every-color-in-the-rainbow tutus, either. She recovered quickly from surgery and tolerated a round of chemotherapy well.

She ran up and down the stairs in Joan's triplex every day, and spent weekends at the house in the country playing with the other dogs, getting around well on three legs. And that's how she lived happily for the rest of her life until the cancer finally won the battle several years later.

When we put Lulu to sleep, Joan cried, and through her tears looked straight in my eyes and said, "I was right to do the surgery. I cannot believe you almost talked me out of it."

What? But then through those same tears, she winked at me. It was Joan's "Thank you."

I tearfully said back, "When you're right, you're right," which was my way of saying, "You're welcome."

I miss that woman daily.

CHAPTER 13

The Secret Lives of Humans

Even if I were a top real estate broker like my client Michele Kleier, I don't think I would have seen the inside of as many Manhattan apartments as I have in my thirty years as a house call vet. We often make visits to more than twelve homes a day, five days a week, fifty-two weeks a year. I have seen a mini-Versailles on the Upper East Side; sleek West Village penthouses ripped from the pages of *Architectural Digest*; Park Avenue townhouses with in-home squash courts; and, of course, lots and lots of homes with museum-quality art and antiques. One eccentric client had a caracal, a lynx-like animal from Africa, wandering around like a house cat.

I've also been inside homes that were so squalid I feared for my health just breathing in the air. The unkempt homes aren't necessarily the ones you think they'll be. Perfectly tidy apartment buildings can hide a hoarder in apartment 3C. And modest apartments in public housing are often as welcoming as any on Fifth

Avenue. I can't predict what I am going to see or hear when I cross a given threshold.

The thing is: I never just pop in. Clients expect me, and the appointments are confirmed and reconfirmed in advance. So it amazes me the things that clients leave out knowing that my nurse and I will be coming over to see their pets. I've seen sex toys, illicit drugs, vials of medications for health problems I certainly wouldn't advertise, dozens of empty wine and liquor bottles lined up on the floor, overdue bills, eviction notices, used condoms hanging from bathroom garbage cans, last week's dirty clothes, and this week's dirty dishes.

It's not that we snoop. The stuff is out in the open. And, often, we need to search an apartment to find a hiding pet. Once we have the patient, we work in whatever room the client designates for us, which is usually the kitchen but sometimes a bedroom. With uncooperative cats, my preference is a small bathroom so they can't get away and hide. And it's been especially in bathrooms that I've seen things that I can't unsee but wish I could.

Why don't clients put their sex toys in a drawer or recycle their empty vodka bottles before we arrive? I have theories. Either they don't care what we see because it's their private space and they'll live in it however they want. Or perhaps it doesn't occur to them that we might notice the bookshelf of porn DVDs. It's also possible that clients simply trust us—as they should—not to expose or judge them for their secrets.

But there is such a thing as *too* much trust. At one Madison Avenue apartment, when the client wasn't home, I worked on a counter right next to three neat stacks of hundred-dollar bills. Clients have left out piles of diamond jewelry and bank statements displaying account numbers and balances. Although it's never been an issue in all my years, I remain concerned that something could go missing on a day that City Pets was there and we might get blamed for it. You'd think savvy New Yorkers would be more careful about their valuables.

Many of my clients are so comfortable with us treating their pets in their absence that they give us their keys or leave one with their doorman for us to use. Sometimes, though, they forget about the access they gave us.

One morning, Shari and I let ourselves into the Sutton Place apartment of a long-term client, a middle-aged man who worked in financial services. He told us that no one would be home, and the doorman gave us the key to let ourselves in. I admit that I didn't shout out, "Hello? City Pets! Is anyone here?" because the client told me he would be at work, as he usually was when I came to treat his shih tzu, Dandy.

Dandy heard us enter and ran to the door. We followed him straight to the kitchen, our usual place to work. Much to our surprise, my client was not at work. Instead, we found him seated at the kitchen table, his pants around his ankles and his laptop open in front of him. He didn't hear us come in because of the loud groaning and slapping sounds coming from his computer—and because he was concentrating hard (as it were) on what he was doing.

His activity stopped abruptly when he saw us standing in the kitchen doorway with our eyebrows up and mouths agape. He dove under the table, and we turned around and walked out. Apologies were unnecessary. He'd obviously forgotten about the appointment, and he had every right to relax in his kitchen or any other room in his own home. When he called to reschedule, he added, "Of course, bill me for that canceled appointment. It was my fault it didn't work out." The story was safe with us.

The Naked Man, as we called him, was a different story entirely. Jared was a freelance writer who was married to a high-powered and huge-salaried corporate executive. It was she who scheduled the appointments for their Siamese cat, Felix, but it was Jared who was home in their West 57th Street apartment for the visits. Jared always answered the door with only a towel around his waist or in tight white briefs no matter what time of day we made the house call.

"Good morning, Jared," I greeted him, keeping my eyes up and on his.

"You're looking well today, Dr. Amy," he replied. "Come on in. Come anytime. Come again and come often." Some variation of this nonsense was his ritual greeting.

I knew he was completely harmless, but having to put up with his off-color and inappropriate remarks was annoying.

"I'll take Felix into the kitchen to do the exam, and you can go put on some clothes," I suggested. He always ignored the offer.

I had my suspicions that his seminudity and passive-aggressive behavior toward my all-female team might be his way of compensating for feeling inadequate to his extremely successful wife. I didn't really care why he did it, I just wished he would stop. It was bad behavior, even in his own home, where we were guests.

Felix was elderly, with medical problems, and so we went often. When he was diagnosed with diabetes and I needed to train the couple on how to do insulin injections, I insisted that both husband and wife be present. Not surprisingly, Jared was fully dressed and quite polite throughout that house call. As I walked in, I couldn't stop myself from saying, "Jared, it's good to see you fully dressed."

His wife seemed confused at first, but when she looked at her husband's rapidly reddening face, she clued in. After we left, Naked Man must have been dressed down by his wife because he never answered the door without pants again.

One of my best clients, a stay-at-home mom of two named Rose, was a woman known for being practical, down-to-earth, and level-headed. She called me one day in an absolute panic about her pet cat, Sophie. At the time, she was staying in her summer home in East Hampton, a beautiful cedar-shingled two-story house with a rear wall of sliding glass doors and a path to the ocean.

"Amy, I'm freaking out! Sophie is missing!" she said through tears. "Someone forgot to close the sliding door to the patio, and she ran away."

She told me the saga of the last five days. As soon as Rose realized Sophie was gone, she and her teenage kids searched the property and went to all their neighbors' houses with photos of the cat. She called the police, and a small army of cops and firefighters combed the area to find Sophie. She hung flyers in town, left bowls of Sophie's food on the patio (the raccoons were thrilled), and put a dirty litter box by the door (this last technique sounds weird but is very effective).

She did everything she was supposed to do, but despite Rose's efforts, there hadn't been a single sighting of Sophie.

"It's been five days," she said, her voice cracking. "I'm worried she's . . ."

"Don't worry. Cats are resilient," I reassured her. "They are born hunters. Even though Sophie is an apartment cat, she's got natural instincts." Of course, those wouldn't help if she were hit by a car or eaten by a larger animal, I knew, but I didn't mention those possibilities.

Rose then said hesitatingly into the phone, "I got the number of a cat psychic. Never in my life have I had my palm read or looked at my horoscope, but I'm so desperate. Should I call?"

"Yes, sure, do it," I said. "You have nothing to lose." I obviously had no confidence in a cat psychic, but anything that gave Rose hope seemed worthwhile.

So Rose called the psychic, one Madame Olga.

Madame Olga was only too happy to help. After her fee was paid by credit card, she began the phone session. "Tell me about Sophie," she said to Rose.

"Well, she's gorgeous," said Rose, welling up. "Long gray hair and tailless with folded down ears. She's a little mischievous, knocking things off the tables. She follows me from room to room. She drinks from the toilet and purrs in her sleep—"

"I have a vision," interrupted Madame Olga. "I see a long road. Is there a long road near your house?"

"Yes! We have a very long driveway!"

"At the end of the driveway, I see a hole," she said. "Go to the hole!"

Rose ran out of the house with her phone, down to the end of the driveway. "There's a sewer opening!" she told the psychic, still on the call. "I can't believe I didn't notice this opening before. I've walked by it a hundred times."

"I feel the cat," said Madame Olga.

Rose got on the ground and tried to peer through the sewer grate, but all she could see was black. She ran back to the house to get some flashlights and returned to the hole with her kids. They shined all the beams into the sewer and sure enough saw two round green eyes reflecting up at them. Rose screamed, "It's her! *It's Sophie!*"

Within minutes, the East Hampton police and the fire departments were back. They pried the sewer grate off and were able to get a ladder down into the hole. A fireman climbed in, and moments later, up he came with poor dirty, mewing Sophie cradled in his arms.

Rose clutched the sludge-covered cat to her chest and said "Thank you, thank you, thank you" a thousand times to the psychic still on the phone, as well as to Sophie's rescuers. The fireman who saved her said, "No problem. This is why I love my job." A local vet checked Sophie out that very afternoon and said she was in pretty good shape, considering she was stuck in a sewer for five days.

Rose called me later that night and told me the whole story. "Can you believe it? The psychic led me right to her. She was so *specific*."

"It's incredible," I genuinely had to agree.

"It worked out, but people are going to think I'm crazy for calling her in the first place. Please don't tell anyone that I called a psychic! I don't want anyone to think of me as a *woo-woo* type."

As secrets go, this one was pretty tame. I said, "Rose, if you're worried what other people think, just don't tell them. Your secret is safe with me. And all that really matters is you got Sophie back."

A couple of years later, Shari and I showed up for a house call at Rose's multimillion-dollar apartment on East End Avenue. It was a regular stop. We went there twice a week to give Sophie a medicated bath for a skin condition she developed unrelated to sitting in sewer sludge for five days.

Rose let me know she'd be out of town for this appointment and that I should just let myself in with the key she'd given me years ago. As usual, Sophie ran in the opposite direction as soon as she heard us come in, but we knew where to look—her spot was under Rose's bed.

But this time we didn't have a chance to find Sophie under the bed because when we walked into the bedroom, we instead found Rose's husband—*in* the bed—with a naked woman.

When he saw me standing in the doorway, he blurted, "Don't tell my wife!"

He did *not* say, "What are you doing here?," "Let me explain!," or even "Get out!" His first instinct was to ask me to lie for him.

For me, this wasn't a close call. I won't lie for somebody, and so when Rose asked me after the visit if everything was normal—as she always did—what was I going to say? *Yes?* No.

I did not keep his secret. I couldn't. Rose soon filed for divorce and got to keep that magnificent apartment—and Sophie.

Too bad she hadn't consulted Madame Olga about her marriage during their cat psychic session.

It's not just what my nurses and I have *seen* that reveals clients' secrets to us. It's also things we've *heard*. Clients often have truly inappropriate or immensely private conversations with me standing right there. They say (or sometimes yell) things they would *never* want a friend or colleague to hear. I've overheard dirty talking to a lover, parents berating their kids, and details of conversations to lawyers (there goes attorney–client privilege). It's tough to take blood while a married couple is having a hissing argument in the next room about in-laws that devolves into ugly character assassination of somebody's mother. It happens all the time.

So why aren't clients more discreet about their lives in my presence? Again, it's probably because they are in their personal space where they feel free to be themselves and rightly feel that in their own homes they don't need to put their "filters" on, even if the City Pets veterinary team is right there.

I was at the home of a regular client, a woman I'll call Mrs. Jones, who was married to one of New York's most prominent businessmen. While I examined her cat, she was deeply involved in a loving, cooing conversation on the phone with a man I presumed was that famous husband, saying things like, "I love you. I can't wait to see you again. I miss you so."

Nice. How lovely that after all these years this married couple is still so romantic!

Mrs. Jones was silent while she listened for a few minutes to the other side's responses and then said, to my surprise, "I am so sorry to hear this, but you're in luck! Dr. Amy is here right now." And she handed me the phone.

I was stunned. *What's going on?!*

"Dr. Amy?" asked the man on the other end. "Ralph is sick."

Ralph? I immediately recognized the voice of a man I will just call Mr. Smith who was also a regular client and also quite married. Ralph was his pit bull.

At the same moment, they both realized that they were busted. They had dropped their guard during their love talk and then rolled right into their worry over Ralph not feeling well. They simply forgot what they had just been up to while I was standing right there.

I told Mr. Smith perfunctorily that I would come by to see Ralph that afternoon and handed the phone back to Mrs. Jones, whose face had gone completely white. None of us ever said another word about it.

A few months later, I was at the home of another client, a very social woman I will call Mrs. Miller, who asked me, "You've worked with Mrs. Jones's and Mr. Smith's pets a long time, right?" I nodded. "Well, I just heard that they both left their spouses for each other! Can you believe it?"

I raised my eyebrows and just shook my head as if in disbelief, then bit my lip and put my head down to treat her dog's ear infection.

I met Malachi Martin early in my career as a young vet working at Park East. Tall, lanky, and dignified, Malachi was an important Irish-born priest with an order on the Upper East Side. In his fascinating life, he had worked at the Vatican with Pope John XXIII, researched the Dead Sea scrolls, was a professor of biblical archeology and paleography, and authored seventeen books, including a bestseller about being an exorcist in Egypt.

I was honored that this man, as charming as he was brilliant, took a liking to me and was a loyal client of mine at Park East. His cairn terrier, Tatianna, seemed to like me a lot, too.

Four days after I was summarily fired from Park East, Malachi heard about it and invited me to lunch at Scalinatella, an Italian restaurant on East 61st Street. Over a glass of wine *before* lunch, he asked, "What are you going to do?"

I said, "It's only been four days since I left, but I think I've already set myself up for now." His face broke into a big grin when I said that.

"Tell me all about where you will be working. Hope it's not too far for me and Tatianna to walk to."

"It's even more convenient for you than Park East," I happily replied. I told him I was going to continue seeing my patients, but in their own homes, which would be remarkably convenient for him. "At Park East, I got to know people pretty well, like I do you. But now that I'm going into people's homes, I think it will be even more personal. That aspect of being a vet is very meaningful to me."

As I said this, Malachi, a man I only knew to be jovial, suddenly looked sad. He grew silent, and at the end of lunch when the coffee came, Malachi said, "My dear Amy, you're incredibly special to me. You're also a very talented veterinarian. Tatty loves you. I love talking with you. But I need you to hear from me that I am going to stay with Park East."

I fully expected Malachi to rejoice at my news and to remain my client, so I was completely thrown by his response. "I don't understand—" I started.

He interrupted, "I have personal reasons. I know that this is for the best."

Genuinely crestfallen, I finished my coffee. Sullenly, we walked out of the restaurant together and said goodbye.

Malachi's rejection really stung. If he cared about me and thought I was such a great person and vet, why then would he stay with Park East? As I walked home, I was upset and confused by his mysterious dismissal, but mainly sad that this joyful, august man was suddenly out of my life. It was indeed the last time we saw each other.

Years later, after Malachi passed away, I was painfully reminded of his death when I saw an obituary notice about him taped on a friend's refrigerator door.

"Did you know Malachi?" I asked her.

She said, "He was a dear friend of my family."

I told her how surprised and hurt I was by his not remaining my client when I started City Pets.

She paused and then said, "Malachi was a complicated man. He was the life partner of my mother's best girlfriend in the world. They lived together."

"But he was a Jesuit priest," I said. "Doesn't that mean he can't . . ." I stopped myself. Now I understood. Malachi had a private, very secret life, and if I'd gone to his home to treat his dog, I would have known more about him than he wanted me to.

I regret to this day that he did not trust me with his secret so that I could at least have had the chance to tell him that his private life wouldn't have affected in the least how I felt about him nor diminished the esteem I had for him.

I've tried not to be fazed by my clients' secrets. But sometimes, despite all that I've seen and heard, I'm still taken by surprise.

Carl Ruderman, a fiftyish dapper man who lived in an elegant townhouse on East 82nd Street, just off Fifth Avenue, had a Cavalier King Charles spaniel. Despite going to his home many times, I didn't know anything about him but assumed he was a lawyer or a banker because he always dressed in three-piece pin-striped suits, a white shirt, Hermès tie, and a pocket square.

After years of care, the Rudermans just stopped calling me. I assumed they found a new vet or moved permanently to Florida, where they wintered.

So, one day in 2018, I was having coffee and paging through Steve's copy of *The Wall Street Journal*, when I noticed Mr. Ruderman's name in an article. The headline: "SEC Accuses Former Playgirl Magazine Owner of Defrauding Investors." The subhead: "Carl Ruderman and 1 Global Capital LLC are accused of fraudulently raising more than $287 million from thousands of investors."*

Clearly, I was *way off* about his being a lawyer or a banker. Turns out, in one facet of his career, Mr. Ruderman was the pub-

---

* Maria Armental and Peg Brickley, "SEC Accuses Former Playgirl Magazine Owner of Defrauding Investors," *Wall Street Journal*, August 29, 2018, www.wsj.com/articles/sec-accuses-former-playgirl-magazine-owner-of-defrauding-investors-1535588221.

lisher of porn magazines *High Society, Climax, Celebrity Skin,* and *Playgirl,* as well as an extremely lucrative phone sex company. Unlike my client Al Goldstein, Mr. Ruderman was a stealth pornographer. He was known in the industry as "the Invisible Man" for keeping his empire a secret from his high-society friends in both Manhattan and Miami.

The Securities and Exchange Commission was investigating him for other reasons. He'd been running a Ponzi scheme and had hoodwinked 3,600 investors in forty-two states for years, conning them out of hundreds of millions to fund his lavish lifestyle of luxury cars, vacations, and multimillion-dollar houses in New York and South Florida—and, one has to assume, veterinary house call appointments.

My very own Bernie Madoff.

CHAPTER 14

The Uber Rich Really Are Different

When I first started working as a young vet in Manhattan, I thought a million dollars was a lot of money and entitled you to be called "rich." I soon learned from my clients that you weren't rich unless you had $10 million in the bank. Then, as both my clientele and insight grew, I realized rich—wealthy—in New York really meant something like *$100 million* in the bank, not just net worth.

But I also learned that it doesn't matter how rich or famous you are. Most of us are the same when it comes to being a pet owner. You could have Monets on the wall and Oscars on the shelf, but if your cat has diarrhea, all you want to talk about is poop. As it should be.

That said, the uber wealthy *are* sometimes baffling in their behavior, and it's taken me a long time to learn not to be put off by their quirks. The vast majority of my clients are gracious and treat me like a respected professional, like they would a people doctor or a lawyer. But a minority of them—nearly always in the category of the superrich—have not been quite as respectful as I would like.

My first appointment of the day was with a billionaire family that lived in a super-skinny skyscraper on East 57th Street. We checked in at the front desk—more like a hotel than a residence—and instead of being directed to the regular elevator bank, the client wanted us to use the service car. We were escorted out of the building and around the corner to the service entrance, where contractors' equipment and the garbage were stacked and transported. The service elevator took us skyward to the sixtieth floor, where it opened into a sprawling kitchen. I assumed I'd do the exam on the 150-pound Saint Bernard there, since I usually work in kitchens, though a bit disappointed I wouldn't get to see more of this *Succession*-worthy apartment.

The housekeeper grunted in our direction, "This way."

She took us to another behind-the-scenes space, a tiny laundry room no more than about 10-by-10 feet square.

"The boss says you stay in here."

With me, Jeanine, our equipment, and the massive dog, we barely had room to turn around. When we finished the exam, the housekeeper yelled at us because all her freshly washed laundry now smelled like dog.

Some of my wealthiest clients delay paying their bills, no matter how small, for as long as they can. When I first started the practice, I tried to get payment at the time of service, like an appliance repairman does. One time, after wrestling with an uncooperative German shepherd on the floor of a Fifth Avenue penthouse for half an hour, I told the client how much she owed me. She reached into her $30,000 red crocodile Birkin bag, pulled out her $1,000

Gucci wallet, and said, "Shoot, I'm completely broke! Can I pay you next time?"

On our way out, I overheard her calling Lutèce, a famous—and famously pricey—French restaurant, to confirm her reservation for that evening for a dinner that probably would cost ten times the amount she couldn't pay me.

Some of my wealthy clients simply forward my bill to their money managers, a process that often sends it into a black hole, never to be seen again even when I ask. "I'm so sorry, it must have gotten lost in the processing. Can you send your bill again?" is not an unusual refrain from those with more money than a bank.

Some even have elaborate schemes to avoid paying.

Valerie, the vampy second wife of one of the most successful Italian restaurateurs in Manhattan, had several dogs in my care. I was at her West Side apartment often, and each time she paid me in cash. Paying in cash was unusual, even years ago, and I wondered if perhaps she was given an allowance by her new husband whose restaurant empire was cash only. We could always count on replenishing the City Pets' petty cash box after her visits without having to go to the bank.

One day, she said, "You know, you've been here three times this month. It's getting expensive. I was thinking we could set up a barter."

I immediately assumed she meant veterinary service in exchange for meals at one of her husband's delicious Italian restaurants since I couldn't imagine what else she had to trade, and so said, "I'd love to!"

From then on, whenever she called me to treat her dogs, I kept track of how much I would have charged for the service and always let her know the amount. After several months, that number was $2,500, which would be a lot of pasta!

Conveniently, I was reciprocating with Al Goldstein for his fun brunch by taking him out to dinner, and because he was a big fan of Valerie's husband's restaurant, I thought that the barter with Valerie would work out perfectly.

I called her and said, "It's time to call in my marker. Can you book me a table for four at the restaurant next Saturday night?"

She said, "That's not going to be possible. Saturday is our busiest night. Can't you do it on Tuesday, Wednesday, or Thursday?"

I was a little shocked by her reply. *Midweek?* When she called for an appointment for one of her dogs, I never said, "It's my busiest day and so I can't make it." I persisted, and she reluctantly agreed to get us in on Saturday.

When we arrived at the restaurant with Al and his date, I said to the maître d', "We are guests of Valerie." I didn't give him a wink, but I thought I made myself clear that the owner's wife was covering our bill. I assumed she'd told the maître d' that we were coming.

The four of us had a fantastic meal and a great time. Al, an eater, enjoyed the baked clams, Caesar salad, huge family-style chicken parm, baked ziti, fabulous wines, and their signature chocolate bread pudding for dessert. We'd just scraped our plates clean when, much to my surprise, the waiter brought a bill to the table . . . for $800!

I didn't understand why we were given a bill at all and wasn't sure how to handle it. So, I left $200 in cash as a tip and signed my name at the bottom of the check. Our party left, full bellied, a bit tipsy, and happy.

We were halfway down the block when the waiter chased me down the street.

He caught my arm and said, "Ma'am, you didn't pay the bill."

I said, "I signed it. We're guests of Valerie."

"Who are you talking about? I don't know who that is."

"Ask your boss. He knows what's going on."

And then we kept walking. I was mortified to have had that scene in front of our guests, as well as now feeling uneasy about the whole transaction. Did Valerie forget to tell the restaurant about our bill? I assumed it would all get straightened out with a phone call in the morning.

The next day, Valerie called me first thing. She was furious, and I was shocked.

"What the hell is wrong with you?" she shouted. "You didn't pay your bill last night!"

I said, "Whoa, whoa, whoa. I didn't pay my bill last night because we bartered for it. You owe me $2,500, and I spent only $800 at the restaurant. And you should know, I left a really generous tip."

"The barter was just to get you a reservation!" she yelled. "It wasn't for the cost of the meal!"

Huh? Okay, I suppose we should have made the terms of our barter explicit, but who in their right mind would trade thousands of dollars in professional services just to be able to get a reservation at a restaurant? It wasn't *that* popular a restaurant, and I surely could have made my own reservation. I called her precisely so she would arrange for them not to give me a bill but to spend some of the money I had on account by not giving her any bills. Yet, she called and berated me each of the next four days for not paying the bill, insisting that I had to.

Sensing that the harassment wasn't going to stop, on the fifth day I made an appointment with the restaurant owner himself. I explained why I hadn't paid the bill and learned from him that

Valerie had never even told him about our barter setup. What's more, it turns out that whenever she had an appointment with me, she got a thousand dollars in cash from her husband to pay me. He now figured out she instead spent that money on cocaine.

I never paid the restaurant bill, and they never paid me. I got stiffed for $1,700. And worse, I won't go back to that delicious restaurant. But New York has so many great Italian places—and so many honest clients—I can live with both losses.

A very eccentric client, Mr. Melvin, often volunteered that he had been a big-time movie producer in Hollywood before retiring and relocating to the Upper West Side in Manhattan. He doted on his two cats, named Reggie and Veronica.

One Saturday night around nine, my service got in touch with me about an "absolutely urgent" call from him. I phoned him right back and asked, "How can I help?"

"You need to come over here right away," he said. "Reggie just scratched me, and he needs to have his nails trimmed. It has to be in the next hour because I want to go to bed at ten."

Was he for real? "I'm sorry," I said, "but I don't make house calls to trim nails on a Saturday night."

After ten seconds of phone silence, he said slowly, "You know, in Hollywood, nobody *ever* said no to me." Plainly, he was used to getting what he wanted when he wanted it.

Though I believed him, I nonetheless replied, "Well, you're in New York now. Here we say no when we should. I'm happy to put you on the schedule for Monday morning. Okay?"

Another long pause. "Fine," he said, and hung up.

This wasn't the last time he made an unreasonable demand on me, and it also wasn't the last time he heard the word "no" from me. We waged this polite war over boundaries for the entire ten years I was his vet. I actually think he enjoyed it. I didn't.

A Fifth Avenue doyenne, Mrs. Beach, called me in a panic one afternoon because she couldn't find her sapphire ring, a family heirloom. "What should I do?" she asked.

Sometimes clients casually asked me advice about non-pet re-lated things, like who is my favorite tailor or dry cleaner, and I always had an answer to those queries. But this one baffled me. "I'm sorry, I just don't know," I said. "Maybe retrace your steps? I once misplaced my engagement ring and frantically searched for it in my apartment. I finally found it under my pager, which had vibrated itself across my night table and ended up on top of the ring."

Mrs. Beach was not amused by my story. "I don't need Nancy Drew. I need a veterinary surgeon."

A surgeon? What is going on here? "You have me at a loss . . ."

Sighing impatiently, she said, "I think Tricky ate my ring. I need you to operate on her right away and get it."

Tricky was her five-year-old West Highland white terrier, a known eater of nonfood items. If she'd really consumed a sap-phire ring, it probably wasn't an alarming development because a ring was unlikely to perforate her stomach or small intestine or do any serious harm.

I said, "I understand your urgency. But there are things we have to do before we operate. First, we need to confirm that Tricky really did eat your ring. A metal object will be visible on an X-ray."

"Why waste time?" she asked. "I don't want the ring damaged by all those fluids and things. *Just operate, I know it's inside Tricky.*"

"I completely understand why you'd want me to operate. But I would need to first locate the ring to know where in her body to retrieve it. I'm sure you don't want me to just start cutting into Tricky's belly randomly. Right?"

She said impatiently, "Just get on with it."

I met Mrs. Beach and her dog at the hospital and rushed the terrier into radiology for an X-ray. I tried to explain the process to the client—first, we'll take pictures from all sides, then develop the film, and finally examine the images on a light box. "It'll take about fifteen minutes," I told her.

She groaned as if I'd said fifteen *hours*. "Please, just get on with it!"

Sheesh, this woman is rude. In the end, the X-ray process took less than ten minutes. The pictures clearly showed the outline of the most enormous ring I had ever seen. The stone itself doesn't show up on the film, but the ring's multipronged setting was wide enough to hold a robin's egg. I guessed the sapphire was upward of twenty carats! And at the moment, it was halfway through Tricky's colon.

Finding it at the *end* of her GI tract was a relief. It'd gotten through the esophagus, stomach, the small and large intestines unobstructed. I shared the good news with Mrs. Beach. "Because of the ring's location in the digestive tract, surgery won't be necessary. She'll pass the ring by herself. We can speed that process along if you'd like."

"No!" she shouted at me. "*You're not listening to me.* I don't want the ring in there one second longer than it has to be."

"Surgery comes with real risks to Tricky. I strongly recommend letting nature take its course. The colon can accommodate a ring that size—"

"Exactly! The colon! *Doctor . . . I . . . do . . . not . . . want . . . my . . . sapphire . . . ring . . . stewing . . . in . . . a . . . mess . . . of . . . dog . . .*

poop! Do you understand me? If you don't operate on her *right now*, I will take her to someone who will."

I blinked at this woman, stunned by her skewed priorities. The ring was already "stewing" in the dog's bowel. Getting it out now or letting it exit on its own wouldn't matter one bit. But she was demanding I do an unnecessary surgery on her dog.

At that moment, George came into the room with a balled-up paper towel. "I think this is what you're looking for," he said.

I opened up the paper towel and saw the *ginormous* sapphire ring. It was as big as an eyeball. And it was only partially cleaned up, streaked with fecal matter.

Tricky had moved fast. She didn't want the surgery, either.

You'd think the client would be happy to see her precious bauble. "Oh my God! *It's disgusting!*" she said, covering her mouth.

Without being asked, George wryly injected, "Tricky is doing fine, by the way."

"Can you clean that up?" Mrs. Beach demanded. "I may never wear that again," she said to herself.

We disinfected and cleaned the ring and gave it back to Mrs. Beach, who received it with two remotely extended fingers as if it were still covered in excrement. I have no idea if she ever wore it again. I surely would have worn it and told anyone who asked the story of its long journey into darkness and back into the sparkling light.

On the other hand, I've also had some uber-rich clients who show a complete disregard for precious objects in order to accommodate the whims of their pets.

Every three weeks I went to see a ten-year-old Siamese cat named Itchy to give him his dose of chemotherapy for intestinal lymphoma. I had to go through the center hallway to reach the elevator to get to the third floor. This was one of my favorite client homes to visit, not because it was decorated to my taste and I wanted to live there, but because on the wall in that center hall hung a huge Van Gogh painting. I stared at the painting each time as I walked past it to the elevator. Viewing rarely seen great art is a perk of my house call experience.

On one visit my client requested that I keep Itchy in the bathroom with the door closed when I was through with his treatment. As I walked down the wide staircase to the entrance hallway, I realized the reason for Itchy's incarceration. My client was exercising her parakeet, Prankster, who was flying from one end of the room to the other when he saw me and landed—right on top of the frame of the Van Gogh. I guess I made him nervous. But then to my horror he lifted his tail feathers and produced a small mound of gray-white pudding poop that plopped right on the front of the canvas in a small dripping smear. Right on the painting. The Van Gogh. I gasped.

"Prankster just pooped on the Van Gogh!" I blurted.

"Oh, don't worry, Prankster does that all the time," said my client. She then casually called to the kitchen for the housekeeper to bring a cloth and the Fantastik. "We just wipe it off," she explained.

Some uber-rich clients, especially those with their own Van Goghs, don't even think the rules apply to them.

Gordon Getty, the billionaire heir of oil baron J. Paul Getty, and his wife, Ann, called me to come to their Fifth Avenue apartment to vaccinate their cats before relocating, I assumed, to San Francisco, where I knew they had a mansion. I'd read about their legendary dinner parties for eighty, which often included an entire company from a Broadway musical to perform. The Gettys were unique billionaire clients. They were deeply involved in the arts and sciences, collected antiques and paintings, founded a book publishing house, and built museums. And they loved to travel. In fact, they owned a Boeing 727 for jet-setting to Nepal, Japan, or wherever.

When George and I entered their apartment that day, we were kind of disappointed because most of their possessions were already packed for the move. There was, however, one small, framed painting leaning against the wall, not yet boxed. I looked at George and said, "Is that a Van Gogh? Does everyone have a Van Gogh now?"

We dared to take a closer look and found the distinct "Vincent" signature I'd seen on paintings in museums. "Do you think anyone would notice if we slipped it into our wheelie?" I asked.

"The statute of limitations on art theft is lifetime," he cautioned. "So not a good idea."

"Why on earth do you know that?" I asked.

Before he could answer, Ann Getty swept in, chic and yet outdoorsy, in slacks and a white blouse, her trademark brunette curls in a cute ponytail. Gordon joined soon after, wearing jeans and a sweater, with salt-and-pepper hair and a permanent smile. Looking at him, you'd have no idea that he was listed in *Forbes* as one of the world's richest people.

They brought us their cat, and I started my physical exam on top of a cardboard packing box in the front foyer. George prepared the vaccinations.

While speaking with the couple, I learned that they were relocating to England, not San Francisco. "I wish I had known that. You might have a problem," I said. "These vaccinations are insufficient to get your cat into England. They have a complicated animal importation process. You need international travel papers, or your cat will have to go into quarantine." The quarantine laws in England have since changed, but back then, it was an ordeal, cumbersome and unpleasant for everyone, particularly the pets.

Ann said, "It won't be a problem."

"You need to have papers just to put your cat on the plane," I said.

Gordon said, "We're flying on our own jet."

"Even then, immigration officials will come onboard your private jet to check your papers when you land."

"But they won't see the cat," said Ann, with a grin. "We'll keep him locked in the bedroom."

They were going to smuggle their cat into England by hiding him in the king-sized bedroom of their private jet.

See, that just would not have occurred to me.

Some of my clients think of me as their friend as well as their veterinarian. That was the case with Jessica, who sometimes shared a lot of personal information with me during my house calls. She lives in an enormous duplex on the Upper East Side with park views and travels in high-society circles. Sitting on the board of several major New York City arts organizations with her wealthy friends, she leads the carefree life of one who has little to worry about.

No matter what time of day I went to her home—never before noon—to see her Persian cats, Jessica greeted us with a meticulous hairdo, full makeup, jewelry, and always wearing baby doll pajamas that barely covered her frame. The diaphanous material left nothing—*nothing*—to the imagination. I have only seen her fully dressed in photographs, like the one in *The New York Times* Style section taken at a fundraiser for the public library. She was wearing a very deep V-neck top with hot pink sequined pants. And why not? She has a Jennifer Coolidge style that makes her look glamorous and sexy. You can tell that her style gives her joy, and that makes her a delight to be around.

I saw her "closet" a few times. It was a 20-by-30-foot bedroom with floor-to-nearly-ceiling clothing racks built in. The racks were filled with brightly colored high-end designer clothing. The emphasis was pink, and many had some kind of embellishment, like sequins or feathers. And to my dismay, there was a separate closet for fur coats.

One day, I went to see Claudius, one of her Persians, who wasn't feeling well. I did routine blood work and found his kidney levels were elevated.

With the lab results in hand, I called Jessica the next day and said, "I want to do an abdominal ultrasound to visualize his kidneys and also get a sterile urine specimen."

Jessica said, "Anything, of course." She, like most of my very wealthy clients, usually simply said, "Do what you have to do; cost is no object," and meant it.

I submitted the urine analysis and the urine culture, and it came back with confirmation of a very unusual bacteria.

"Claudius has an infection," I told Jessica. In an ideal world I would do blood and urine tests on all my elderly patients every six months so I could preemptively find things like kidney changes or infections before the patients get ill.

I told her Claudius needed medication, and with her booming voice, she practically shouted, "Dr. Amy, do what you need to do," into the phone. I began his antibiotic treatment.

A few days later, Jessica called again. "After your last house call, I realized I hadn't had *my own* blood checked in a while. So, I did it, and just found out that my kidney values are elevated, too.

It gets even weirder. They cultured my urine. And it turns out, I also have bacteria in my urine."

Hmmm. Could it be the same bacteria as her cat? "We need to pursue this. I'm sending you Claudius's culture results for you to show to your doctor.

She called again a few days later. "I wish you were my doctor because you explain things so much better. My bacteria *are* the same as the cat's. He doesn't think that I gave the bacteria to him or that Claudius gave it to me. What do you think?"

Pure coincidence? "If it were me, I wouldn't ignore this. It's probably good to use extra precaution when cleaning the litter pan and consider not sleeping with him until this is resolved."

Neither of their kidney values ever returned to normal, her doctor didn't pursue it and so we never solved the medical mystery of where those identical bacteria came from, or whether they transmitted them to each other. Maybe it came from Jessica's genuine emu-feathered boas?

On a subsequent visit, this time for Jessica's Persian cat, Antony, she welcomed me into the kitchen in her trademark transparent baby dolls. A well-dressed man was already in the kitchen, seated at the large glass table where I usually work. I watched as he pulled out four large black velvet trays and began placing heavy gold bracelets on them.

"Amy, I'm glad you're here. I'm going to need your opinion," said Jessica. "This is Mr. Bravos from LALAoUNIS. I'm thinking of buying some jewelry from him," pointing to the glittering array of gold he was setting up on the table.

Mr. Bravos probably brought those trays in a suitcase handcuffed to his wrist from the elegant shop on Madison Avenue. I passed the store every day when I worked at Park East and often stared in the window at the beautiful baubles thinking, *One day, one of you will be mine.*

I *love* the Greek fine jewelry brand LALAoUNIS. I adore their use of imagery from ancient history in their designs, like Hellenic knots and mythological figures. You could easily imagine every necklace, ring, bracelet, and pair of earrings being worn by Hera or Aphrodite. Perhaps I was drawn to the pieces because my dad's family was Greek, but more likely it was because they're just so beautiful. The work was expertly crafted with the most magnificent quality jewels and metals.

And I do have a special relationship with a LALAoUNIS necklace.

In 2010, the Veterinary Medical Association of New York City bestowed on me the Award for Outstanding Service to Veterinary Medicine. I would receive the award at a black-tie gala, emceed by Jon Stewart. Even though I was thrilled to be so honored, the event came at a sad time for us as Steve's dad had recently passed away. Despite his grief, Steve told me, "Your peers are honoring you, and so we're going to make it a special evening. Let's go to Bergdorf Goodman and buy the most beautiful gown in the world." We went together to this extraordinary one-of-a-kind department store and chose a gorgeous, sexy red chiffon gown by the timeless designer Vicky Tiel.

The night of the gala, after I was fully dressed, I opened the little safe in my bedroom closet where I kept my jewelry to retrieve the pearl necklace I was planning to wear. Right in front, I found a beautifully wrapped gift box with a Post-it note on it that read: *Wear me tonight.*

Breathless, I opened the box and found a magnificent necklace from LALAoUNIS! It was perfect for my gown's neckline, and the

Hellenic design incorporated little rubies that were the same color as the dress.

Delighted, I ran to my husband, "Steve! What have you done?"

He told me how he'd gone to every jewelry store—from Harry Winston to Cartier—with a photograph of me in my Vicky Tiel gown and a swatch of the fabric, to find the right piece to wear with my new gown. His last stop was LALAoUNIS, where he struck gold (literally) and found the perfect necklace to go with the dress.

So when I found Mr. Bravos and his displays of LALAoUNIS designs on Jessica's kitchen table, I felt all the emotions of that time. My one beautiful necklace represented my husband's love and being honored by my colleagues. Very special.

Jessica was picking through the display, piece by piece, her generous bosom propped on the counter next to the trays as if they, too, were on offer. She tried on everything. She focused on two large, bejeweled cuff bracelets of pure gold. They were similar, as each bracelet closed with large medallions, one with a lion's head and the other with a ram's head. Rubies, emeralds, sapphires, and diamonds were abundantly but tastefully used to highlight the animal's facial expression.

"Amy, which one do you prefer?" she asked me. "Do you like this one?" She tried on the lion's head cuff, and then the ram. She didn't wait for me to answer. She said to Mr. Bravos, "I don't know. I'm thinking . . . They're both beautiful . . . I can't make up my mind. Fine, I'll take both."

Watching this casual decision to buy multiple pieces of expensive jewelry from the very jeweler my husband had turned to for a once-in-a-lifetime event made me wonder, If it is so easy and you have so much, is it possible to really appreciate it all?

I was at the home of a well-known Manhattan plastic surgeon to examine Chowder, the family's Cavalier King Charles spaniel, who had heart disease. As usual, I placed Chowder on the kitchen table. This kitchen was the stuff of any chef's dreams. It had a Viking double oven, a glass door Sub-Zero fridge, two dishwashers, and a bunch of other appliances I didn't even recognize. You could cook anything in this kitchen. But in the five years I'd been coming here, I had never once seen anyone prepare food, much less even turn on one of those machines.

That evening, my client—dressed elegantly in Armani, her favorite designer—and I were talking about Chowder's health when her daughter whined loudly from another room, *"Mommm! When's dinner? I'm starvinnng!"*

My client yelled right back, "Dinner's almost ready!"

Dinner's almost ready? Nothing was happening in the kitchen I was standing in other than a veterinary house call. The client turned to me and said, "Excuse me for just one second." She went to the wall phone, hit a speed-dial button, and said in an exasperated voice, "Hello? Le Bernardin? I called with a dinner order *forty-five minutes ago* and it's not here yet."

Le Bernardin is one of New York's few three-Michelin-starred restaurants. You need to make reservations there months in advance and should expect to pay the equivalent of your Manhattan rent for a single meal. And she had the place on her *speed dial*. For delivery. *For her teenager's dinner on a Wednesday.*

I finished with Chowder before the food arrived so I will never know if a uniformed butler delivered it. I went home and reheated leftovers.

❖

Some of the uber rich even create their own reality. This was true of Ivana Trump, a client I first met when I was at Park East. At that time, she had just survived a scandalous, front-page divorce from her first husband, Donald J. Trump, and was perhaps the most famous and glamorous single mother in America.

She came to Park East with her black poodle, Choppy, who had a broken leg. I was not the first vet she consulted about Choppy. In her Czech-accented English, she said, "All doctors tell me put pins and metal plates in leg. They don't know anything. I was professional skier and I know. Putting pins in Choppy vill ruin his life."

I agreed with the other vets she'd spoken to. Choppy was young, and surgical repair was the right thing to do for him. The ends of the bones needed to be aligned and fixed in the proper position for him to heal properly. But this was not what she wanted to hear so she went elsewhere for a leg cast.

She didn't call me again for years. By then, Choppy was elderly, with a lot of medical issues. She called because he was coughing excessively. He had a heart murmur, other signs of heart disease, serious dental problems including loose teeth, and severe arthritis.

She said to me, "So vat is wrong vid him? Vhy does he cough so much?"

I went through the list of his problems and highlighted the heart issues. "He needs a chest X-ray and an echocardiogram, and once his cardiac issues are sorted out, he will need to have a proper dental. I can also put him on medication for his arthritis."

She nodded, and I thought, *Her bouffant does not actually move.*
She said, "Thank you."
She never called for a follow-up.

The next time Ivana called, it was years later for her cat Koshka. I went to her five-story limestone townhouse on East 64th Street, ironically, just down the block from Park East Animal Hospital. Her assistant met me in the vermillion and gold lobby where I waited for my patient.

Mrs. Trump swanned down the grand marble staircase wearing a long caftan and ballet flats, carrying an obese cat. She said to the air, "Koshka has green coming out of eyes."

I took possession of the cat when she landed. "Okay. Let me take a look at him. Where shall I do the exam?" I asked.

"Through here," said Ivana, pointing to a door that led to a much less glamorous staircase to the building's basement.

Sadly, I never got to go upstairs to see the cheetah-themed den, the pink marble double bathroom, the white grand piano in the living room, daughter Ivanka's childhood bedroom with a four-poster bed and canopy, or the gown closet I'd heard Ivana called "Indochine" because it was so long that by the time you got to the end you might as well be on another continent. All I got to see was the dank basement. I found a clean-enough table, examined the cat, and found that he had severely dry eyes. I explained to her, "He's going to need multiple eye drops, probably for the rest of his life, to treat this condition."

"Okay, good. Thank you so much," she said, ever polite.

She never filled the prescriptions. She never called again.

I'll never know what she was thinking. She called when her pets had problems, but she didn't follow up on the proper treatments. And just another example of how the uber rich really are different.

CHAPTER 15

Who's the Patient Here?

Good doctoring is so much more than administering pills and giving injections. Especially for veterinarians, it requires careful observation, since our patients are unable to describe their symptoms. As a result, there are times a veterinarian observes the client as well as the pet and realizes that the human is in need, too. I have been the recipient of a veterinarian's medical care, and I have been known to help a human or two while vetting their pets.

When Bumper, my elderly blind pug, was suffering from severe arthritis and was no longer responding to traditional treatment, I decided to try alternative therapy. I called my colleague and old friend veterinarian Allen Schoen. Allen was one of the first to specialize in alternative forms of care and had written the veterinary book on acupuncture. I'd known him for years—my freshman-year biology professor had introduced me to him. Allen was his college roommate and now was attending veterinary school at Cornell. Allen and I corresponded for a long time but didn't actually meet until we were both working at the Animal

Medical Center years later. Allen eventually set up his own clinic about ninety minutes north of the City, and it was there that I referred my patients for acupuncture. I even sent Valerie, the restaurateur's wife who stiffed me, with one of her dogs. (I wonder if she tried to barter with Allen for a free dinner reservation?)

At one of Bumper's treatments, Allen looked at me while inserting the acupuncture needles into my dog and said, "Amy, you don't look well. Are you feeling okay?"

"As a matter of fact, I'm not," I said. "I'm getting the aura that always comes before a migraine. I don't know when it's going to start. If it hits me on the way home, I'm not going to be able to drive." The thought of being incapacitated on the highway with Bumper in the car was stressing me even more. Bumper, however, was unfazed, as he was sleeping and snoring loudly, as he always did during his treatments even though he had eighteen acupuncture needles in him.

The stress of my new house call practice seemed to be worsening my migraines. To combat them, my doctor kept increasing the dosage of medicine, which wasn't working but was instead making me incredibly tired during the day. It got so bad that I often wanted to go home and nap in the middle of a busy day.

Allen asked, "Do you mind if do some acupuncture on you?"

I'd never had acupuncture before, but I knew how much relief Bumper got from it. I immediately agreed.

Allen used his fingers to massage acupressure points on my forehead and the back of my neck. Within minutes, the aura stopped, and I felt better. I drove back home, still bracing for the migraine to come, but it never did. After the acupressure (and for the first time ever), the aura wasn't followed by the splitting headache.

I'd gone to Allen for Bumper but ended up getting treatment myself.

That impromptu acupressure session changed my life. I began to see an acupuncturist in the City twice a week. On the first visit, he placed the needles one by one, and the next thing I knew, I was being woken up from a very deep sleep a half hour later. For the rest of that day, I felt great. Within two months, I was off all migraine medications, and migraines are no longer a problem for me.

Like Allen, the work I do doesn't begin and end with the animals. When I see suffering, my impulse is to heal. I go to my clients' homes to treat their cats and dogs, but I have treated the humans as well. Sometimes my clients become my "patients."

Patsy Cline Jacobson, a feisty calico cat, lived on the fifth floor of a small, no-elevator brownstone on the Upper West Side. I knew those stairs well; I had been climbing them with my equipment monthly for a very long time. Patsy Cline had advanced kidney disease along with many of its complications. Priscilla, her owner, often described the cat as "all I have in the world."

George and I cursed each time we carried a month's worth of supplies up those stairs, including large heavy bags of sterile electrolyte fluids that we taught Priscilla to inject into Patsy Cline every day. At eighteen and a half, the cat was no longer responding to the treatments, and she was a frail shadow of her former self. She didn't interact with Priscilla and had stopped eating and cleaning herself. I tried several times to discuss humane euthanasia with Priscilla, but she covered her ears when I brought up the subject.

On my final visit to see Patsy Cline, Priscilla had to listen. The cat was lying on her side, semiconscious and gasping for breath. My quick assessment confirmed that she was dying, although I didn't know if it would happen swiftly or peacefully. I sat with Priscilla and explained that she didn't have a choice.

"Patsy is suffering," I said bluntly. "She is unable to breathe and if I don't put her to sleep, she might suffer for hours."

Priscilla looked spacey herself while I spoke, so I made her repeat back to me exactly what I told her. Eventually, she agreed that I should put Patsy Cline to sleep. Within seconds of giving Patsy the euthanasia solution, she peacefully passed. I confirmed this by placing my stethoscope on her heart. There was no longer a heartbeat.

"Is she gone?" Priscilla asked through sobs.

I nodded and whispered, "Yes. She is."

Priscilla continued sobbing, then threw herself to the ground, lay on her stomach, and began banging her fists and feet on the floor in a tantrum.

"I don't want to live anymore!" she screamed between sobs. "I want to die, too."

I'd never seen a reaction like this. Although I didn't know exactly what to do, I knew that I could not leave her alone. I had to take her shouts of "I don't want to live" seriously, but I am not trained to help people who were this distraught. I needed help.

I had an idea. I asked George to stay with Priscilla, and then I walked around the small apartment opening cabinet doors. In the bathroom medicine cabinet, I found what I was looking for. There were several vials of pills that I recognized as antipsychotic medications. I knew that looking in her medicine cabinet was a violation of her privacy, but given the situation, I felt it was medically necessary.

The prescribing doctor's name and phone number were on the

pill vials. Using Priscilla's home telephone, I called his office and explained to the receptionist that I had an emergency with one of his patients.

The psychiatrist came to the phone immediately and I told him what happened. He asked to speak with her, and I pulled the land-line cord as far as it could go to get Priscilla on the call. He spoke to her for several minutes until she was calmer. She sat up and continued to have a conversation with her doctor. She looked drained but at last was behaving more normally.

I was still reluctant to leave her alone. We waited until she was calmer, although still crying, and then left with Patsy Cline.

I called Priscilla's psychiatrist one more time that day and al-though he couldn't discuss her case with me, he assured me that she would be all right now.

I never heard from Priscilla again. Perhaps she never got an-other cat so didn't need me. But I think about her often as a re-minder to me of human fragility to which, sometimes, I bear witness and, occasionally, provide some care.

Mr. Melvin, my retired, bossy movie producer client, who was now in his seventies, still had his two cats, Reggie and Veronica. He and his wife, a former mezzosoprano, lived in an apartment on the forty-third floor of a modern building near Lincoln Center. I don't remember ever meeting Mrs. Melvin, because she was at work during the day and often traveled with her opera company.

Reggie, a gray tabby, needed monthly steroid injections for his severe inflammatory bowel disease. Over the years, Mr. Melvin had become agoraphobic—having a fear of leaving home—so he was always there for our visits. He still liked to think he was in his high-powered career, and he continued to bark orders to everyone, us included. George and I called him "Mr. Apple" because at the end of our visits, he always offered us a Granny Smith, befitting his sour demeanor perhaps. George always ate it.

I was dreading my upcoming visit with him because I knew that Mrs. Melvin had been on tour for a while and that always put her husband in a bad mood. But when I got to his apartment, Mr. Melvin was strangely passive.

George asked, "Dr. Amy, do you smell that?"

I did. The apartment smelled foul, like an organic chemistry lab.

I have a very sensitive nose. I've gone to clients' homes and noticed a faint gas smell, which led to the discovery of a gas leak in the building, and once, I detected that sewage was seeping into a client's walls. But I don't think anyone could have missed this stench. How could Mr. Melvin stand it? But, then again, because of his condition he never left the apartment. If this odor had gotten stronger slowly over time, it's possible he was not even aware of it. I went to open a window, but I couldn't because in this newly constructed skyscraper, the windows didn't open.

Mr. Melvin could barely respond to questions, and his words were slurred. The odor and his condition were so alarming that we put the cats in carriers and then cajoled him out of the apartment. I'd been inside for less than ten minutes and I was already feeling nauseated.

In the building lobby, I parked Mr. Melvin on a couch, put George in charge of him and the cats, and went in search of the building's superintendent. I found him in his office and told him what was going on. He said, "There are renovations going on next door to his apartment. We've given them notices for months because they're using chemicals that aren't permitted in the building." Apparently, the rooms being renovated were right next door to Mr. Melvin's bedroom, and the notices had no impact on their use of the chemicals.

The super went to Mr. Melvin's apartment and opened all the windows (apparently, he had some kind of tool to do that). Then he went next door and immediately halted the renovations going on there.

Fortunately for Mr. Melvin, Reggie's steroid injections were due just then, and we recognized his confusion and got him out of the apartment. Although he recovered fully, had he been exposed to those chemical fumes much longer he might have suffered brain damage.

The next time we went to that Lincoln Center tower to give Reggie his steroid shot, Mr. Melvin was back to his crotchety old self. He barked orders at us and as usual didn't say thank you for our care of his cat, much less for saving his brain and maybe his life.

But when we were getting ready to leave, he gave us *two* apples.

Although I wasn't eager to go inside Gail the hoarder's East 26th Street one-bedroom apartment to treat her cat, Sweetie, we still went to see her every month or so for many years. At each visit, the place was more crowded and suffocating with food waste, trash, boxes of things she'd found, and higher piles of newspapers, magazines, and other junk. Sweetie navigated the stacks, jumping from one to the next, like Queen of the Mountain. They both seemed content to live like that, but I loathed every minute inside that apartment. It was unsanitary, and even though we put on surgical booties, gloves, and masks, I felt contaminated just being in there.

But I couldn't abandon Gail because she and Sweetie needed

my help. If I didn't go to her, I doubted she'd have the wherewithal to take Sweetie to a brick-and-mortar animal hospital. Besides, I wanted to lay eyes on Gail every few months to check on her health, too. I wasn't giving her an exam, but I did scan her for signs of illness, both physical and mental, at each visit, and snuck in some casual questioning about her habits, such as, "Did you eat today?," "Are you sleeping?," and "Have you been outside recently?"

Meanwhile, the conditions became so bad, it was too unpleasant for me to examine Sweetie inside the apartment. I made an excuse that wouldn't hurt Gail's feelings—I blamed it on my allergies—and said, "From now on, I need to examine Sweetie in the hallway right outside your door."

Gail said, "Okay. It'll give me a chance to do some cleaning up." She hadn't taken the garbage out for months, but apparently today was going to be the day.

While I examined the cat on the hallway floor, Gail started bringing bags of garbage out from her apartment to the trash incinerator chute, which was next to where I was working. As she brought out bag after bag, one of them disintegrated, and liquid detritus poured out the bottom, all over me and my equipment. Everything I had with me now smelled like a Port Authority bathroom. I didn't say anything. Gail was so proud of herself for taking out a small fraction of the trash, I didn't want to discourage her from doing it again. My cleanup would begin when we were done here.

Periodically, I simply called to check up on them. Gail often said, "I'm glad you called. I couldn't find your number and Sweetie isn't feeling well." I had placed refrigerator magnets with my contact information all over her apartment.

I always responded, "No problem, we'll come by today."

I never found anything seriously wrong with the affectionate cat. I think she just wanted company. But the visits gave me an opportunity to check in on Gail's health and wellness as well, and it went on like this for years.

On one visit, there was something wrong. Gail said that Sweetie wasn't acting normally. It was true. Sweetie wasn't right. Her pupils were widely dilated, and they didn't constrict, even when I shined a bright light directly into them. Using a special lens to visualize her retina, I could see that hers had detached from the back surface of her eyes. Sweetie was blind. The most common cause for this was high blood pressure, and Sweetie's pressure was well over 200, which is sky-high for kitties.

I needed to get her blood pressure under control immediately and didn't trust that Gail could medicate her reliably. I brought Sweetie back to the hospital with me, where she was treated and monitored. After three days on medication, her blood pressure normalized, and her retina miraculously reattached. Sweetie was able to see again.

Upon discharge, I explained to Gail, "We have a happy outcome today. But Sweetie's blood pressure will go right back up and she could lose her vision again if you don't give her the medication at the same time every day."

"I hear you," she said. "I'll do it, I swear."

Just like she'd promised to scoop the litter box and swore she would give Sweetie fresh food every day? She meant well, but I also knew she'd forget. I added "Call Gail" to my daily schedule and each morning, I phoned her and asked, "Did you give Sweetie the blood pressure medication?"

Every morning, she said, "I don't have any blood pressure medication."

"Yes, you do. It's in your refrigerator. Go check."

"I don't know what you're talking about . . . Oh, yes, here it is."

Every day, I stayed on the phone until she'd dosed the cat. Every other day, I or one of my nurses went back to Gail's apartment to give the cat fluid injections for her recently diagnosed kidney issues, which Gail simply did not have the capacity to do.

One day, Gail didn't pick up her phone. When we went to the apartment for Sweetie's fluid injection, no one answered the buzzer. I knew something was terribly wrong but didn't know how to find out.

Eventually, I taped a note to the front door of the building addressed to "Superintendent." In it, I explained how worried I was about Gail and Sweetie, wrote down my phone number, and urged him to call me with some news.

An hour later he called. "Is Gail okay?" I asked, my hand went to my heart, fearing the worst.

"Gail had a stroke. She's now in a long-term care facility," he said. "Her family set it up." *She has a family? Where have they been all these years?*

"And where is Sweetie?"

"She's still in the apartment. I go in a few times a day. I give her the medication in the fridge, feed her, and clean the litter pan. I don't know what to do with these fluids, though."

I paid a visit to check on Sweetie and meet the super. I found the cat in good condition and said to him, "She's doing very well with you."

He nodded. "She's a good cat, but I can't keep her."

"Give me a chance to figure out what to do," I said.

Within twelve hours, Shari volunteered to foster Sweetie.

I got in touch with Gail's newfound family and spoke to her niece. She told me that Gail was doing as well as can be in rehab. When she recovered, she would be moving into a nursing home.

The apartment was going to be cleaned out (hopefully by someone in a hazmat suit) and re-rented. It was the end of an era.

I was sad that the independent part of Gail's life was over. She was troubled but content in her own cluttered world with her cherished pet. I believe that if it weren't for the love of Sweetie, Gail wouldn't have been mentally or physically capable of living independently for as long as she did.

"What about Sweetie?" I asked. "She's living with my nurse, who would be happy to keep her."

"I'll take her as soon as the dust settles with Gail," she said. Shari was disappointed but it was the right thing.

The last I heard about Gail and Sweetie was the day when the niece drove to Shari's house to pick up the cat. To this day, I miss them both (but not that apartment).

The first time that I met Mrs. Blum, she told me that she stayed alive only to take care of her eighteen-year-old poodle, Maggie. Many people say things like that, but Mrs. Blum was ninety and quite fragile, and she lived alone without friends or family other than Maggie. Maybe for her, it was true.

I went to her small apartment on First Avenue, and she told me the reason for the appointment. "Maggie hasn't eaten in three days."

I knew immediately that Maggie was very sick. After an examination, I found she was in congestive heart failure and had advanced kidney failure, and the treatment for one disease would exacerbate the other. Maggie was dying, and there wasn't a thing I could do about it.

I wasn't sure Mrs. Blum understood the seriousness of Maggie's problems. Her dependence on her little poodle was total, and I knew that soon Maggie would be gone. I was very worried about what would happen next.

"Please, Dr. Amy. Take her to the hospital and make her better." I agreed to take her to the hospital but was not optimistic that I would be making her better.

Usually, I'm immediately open with clients about their pet's prognosis, no matter how grim. But with Mrs. Blum, I was afraid that the bad news would affect her own health and I had a responsibility both to dog and human.

Maggie was in the hospital for two days and was getting worse. What would be the gentlest way to tell Mrs. Blum what the outlook was for Maggie?

I decided to deliver the news in person, but not alone. I remembered that Mrs. Blum had been an active member of a local church years ago. The priest of the church was coincidentally also my client, and so I called him to ask if he'd go with me to tell Mrs. Blum about Maggie. He remembered her fondly and agreed to join me and lend spiritual support.

This was a good plan. But at the very time I was on the phone with the priest setting things up, Maggie passed away peacefully in her sleep while still in the hospital.

So now we had to go to Mrs. Blum with much worse news.

With the priest at my side, I said, "I'm so very sorry, Mrs. Blum. Maggie had severe heart and kidney failure. She passed away an hour ago. She was asleep and felt no pain, I'm certain of it."

Thank God the priest was with me, because Mrs. Blum immediately became distraught. This frail elderly lady started crying and sank into the couch so deep, it was as if she wanted to disappear.

I had done all I could do as her veterinarian and then stayed as her friend to console her, but now had to leave for other appointments. I felt awful leaving her like this but the priest said that he'd stay for as long as Mrs. Blum needed him to.

I called him several times over the next few days. On the third day he told me, "She won't get out of bed. I'm making sure she eats at least a bite or two, but most of the time, she just lies there and stares at the ceiling."

"That's it?" I asked. "Does she talk with you?"

"Sometimes she cries."

It seemed true that Mrs. Blum had been keeping herself alive just to take care of Maggie. And now that Maggie was gone, what did that mean for Mrs. Blum?

To me, it meant she needed another dog, right away. I know many people need time to grieve for one pet before they get another, but Mrs. Blum didn't have time to wait. She needed a new focus, a new purpose, a new love, immediately.

I called all my dog rescue contacts and put the word out that I needed an older, small poodle with a good temperament who would be happy living indoors in an apartment with a senior citizen. Within a week, I'd located Pierre, an eight-year-old toy poodle.

Excited, I went over to Mrs. Blum's apartment. She answered the door but was completely disheveled, shrunken, and sullen. She was still in her nightgown. It was the first time that I had ever seen her like this.

"Mrs. Blum, I need your help. I have a little poodle. His name is Pierre. His family moved away and just left him. He has no home, and I need someone to look after him. He is in good health. He loves sitting on people's laps and being brushed. He is a very quiet boy. And he has a clean bill of health."

She shook her head sadly and said, "I can't do it. I'm too old to start loving a dog again. And at my age, it wouldn't be fair to the dog."

"I understand. But I am not asking you to keep him. Would you be willing to just meet Pierre?" I asked. "Maybe he can stay here for a few days while I find a home for him? You'd be doing *me* a huge favor."

"Just a few days?" she asked.

Two hours later, I was back at Mrs. Blum's with Pierre. The instant I put him into her hands, Mrs. Blum said to him, "You're so handsome!" and broke into a huge smile. The first smile I'd seen since Maggie went to the hospital. And little Pierre knew exactly what to do. He looked up at Mrs. Blum and licked her face, and he didn't stop licking, all while his tail was going a mile a minute.

I got goose bumps watching them. He'd been so quiet and reserved with me. But, boy, was he happy with her.

Mrs. Blum turned to me and said, "Good thing you brought him here. This dog clearly needs a home."

Yes, he did. And she needed to give him one.

Pierre never left.

Research shows that dog ownership is associated with better health and longevity. Mrs. Blum already had a good long life, but now that she had Pierre to take care of, I hoped I would be seeing both of them for years yet to come, which is just what happened.

CHAPTER 16

A Beginning and Three Endings

Apart from my summer college internship at a dairy farm, I haven't had much experience birthing baby animals. Most of my dog and cat patients are neutered, so they aren't breeding the next generation. And, frankly, I discourage my clients from breeding their pets, urging them to leave that to professional breeders.

Once, I delivered a litter of shih tzu puppies when I was a young vet at Park East. They belonged to my client's teenage daughter, Marie-Chantal, who called my service at 11:30 p.m. because the family's very pregnant shih tzu was starting to act strangely while on her bed.

Long before I even dreamed of being a house call vet, I went to the family's townhouse to assist in this birth. With my help, the mother dog delivered five tiny, mucous-covered, healthy puppies on Marie-Chantal's bedspread. I quickly dried the pups, stimulated them to suckle, and returned each to their mama, who was ready to nurse. Thirty years later, Marie-Chantal—now the crown princess of Greece—is still my client. She has another wonderful pack of dogs.

I do have extensive experience at the other end of life. Deciding with a client when to put a pet to sleep is the most solemn and important duty I have as a vet. It is my job to guide families through this decision. I have done thousands of euthanasias over the years, and they're painful every time.

My first year in practice at AMC, as I put a pet to sleep, I was so moved by a man's loving words to his pet as he said goodbye that tears streamed down my own face. A senior clinician witnessed this and said later that day in an attempt to comfort me, "Don't worry, Amy. Give it a little time, and after doing enough of them, you won't cry during a euthanasia."

I usually appreciated his sage advice, but this time, I thought, *The day I stop crying during a euthanasia, I should no longer be doing this job.* I have never stopped crying.

Michele Kleier lost her Maltese Lily after her yearslong, heroic battles with multiple cancers. But it was worth it for this family to get the extra quality time with their loving pet whom they adored in return. After Lily passed, I hoped Michele's remaining dogs would stay healthy for a while. But that was not to be.

"I'm worried about Daisy," Michele said on the phone one day, speaking of her fourteen-year-old Maltese. "Last night, she jumped up in her sleep, urinated, and then tumbled off the bed onto the carpet. And ever since, she's acting weird and walking funny. Something's going on. She's been a little off for a few days."

I did preliminary tests that were all inconclusive and Daisy's demeanor continued to deteriorate. I sent her to a veterinary neurologist for a consult. He concluded that her behavior was consistent with a central nervous system issue and scheduled her for a brain MRI. A large and inoperable brain tumor was seen on the MRI results. The size and shape of the tumor was consistent with a diagnosis of meningioma. Although this tumor is technically benign, hers had to be treated because it was occupying space within her skull that was needed for her brain, and the mass was already causing her neurologic deficits, which would only get worse as the tumor got larger.

There was only one option to offer Michele for Daisy's treatment, which was daily radiation therapy to her brain. The protocol would be difficult. Each treatment had to be done under general anesthesia. The sessions would be five days a week for at least three weeks. As if that weren't bad enough news, the only hospital we could find that had an appropriate and functioning radiation machine was at Cornell University, all the way upstate in Ithaca, New York, an eight-hour drive from New York City.

Without even a thought, the Kleiers agreed to treatment and devoted themselves to Daisy. Michele and her husband drove the eight hours to Ithaca every Sunday, took Daisy for her five daily radiation treatments at Cornell, and then made the long drive back to the rest of their family in New York City every Friday evening. They upended their lives for a chance to prolong their fourteen-year-old dog's life.

The radiation in fact shrunk the tumor, but she developed complications from the steroids she was taking to control radiation swelling. The steroids caused Cushing's disease, which made her excessively hungry, thirsty, and agitated. And then, three weeks into her therapy, she was accidentally given a double dose of radiation, which caused severe ulcers in both of her eyes.

The treatment was halted, and Michelle was understandably very upset. "Hasn't my poor baby been through enough?" she literally cried to me. We had two weeks to decide what to do, because Daisy's eyes needed to heal before treatment resumed. And then we learned that the radiation therapy unit at Cornell was broken for the foreseeable future.

Michele said to me through tears, "I think the universe is trying to tell me 'no more.' First the tumor, then Cushing's, then the overdose and the ulcers, now the machine is down—and my poor girl is just miserable from all the steroids."

When do you say *stop*?

Most clients say it long before Michele and Ian did. Daisy was sick, but she slept in bed with them, she played with them and kissed them, and she still looked adorable. She was their beloved dog, albeit diminished but seemingly happy to be alive and with her family.

Michele, a rare breed of human, would never consider euthanasia out of convenience or because of the cost of treatment, much less the difficulties it posed for her personally. She proved that again and again with Fluffy, Lily, Daisy, and then Dolly, her next Maltese, who sustained a traumatic brain injury. And after Dolly was Tootsie, the rescue, who developed vasculitis, a narrowing of tiny blood vessels, that caused part of her ear to fall off. Maltese aren't an illness-prone breed, but sadly the Kleiers might be. Michele took such good care of her pack that they lived long enough to have interesting problems.

The treatments, costs, life disruptions, and the angst followed by sadness. Was it worth it? To Michele and her family, yes. Absolutely.

Others might say, "You're just prolonging the inevitable." And they would be right. But prolonging the inevitable is what I do every day. I give vaccines to animals so they don't get sick and give them treatments to help them live longer, healthier lives. In essence, my day job is prolonging the inevitable.

But they all do eventually die, most likely long before we do. We know this as pet owners. The joy of every new pet comes with knowledge of future sadness. And to me, willing acceptance of that knowledge in exchange for the love is proof of the extraordinary bond we have with our animals.

I met Tommy Tune, the legendary Broadway choreographer and dancer, through our mutual friend, Joan Rivers. He had a beloved Yorkie named Ophie. Tommy lived on East 88th Street in an apartment that was designed to accommodate his six-foot-six height.

I couldn't set up like I normally would in his kitchen because Tommy's custom countertop was too high for me to use to examine Ophie. So I usually worked on his couch, which was at an acceptable height. When I finished, someone would bring a small stepladder just so I could reach the kitchen faucet and wash my hands.

Besides feeling like I'd entered the Jolly Green Giant's castle, Tommy's apartment was bright, fun, and theatrical. The navy carpeting throughout the apartment had little gold stars woven into it that looked like the Hollywood Walk of Fame.

On one visit, the carpet was covered with masking tape in straight lines and arrowheads. One pointed left into a bathroom, and another right into a guest room.

"Tommy, what's with the tape on the carpet?" I asked.

"Carol Channing is staying with me and sometimes she can't find her way from the bedroom to the bathroom," he said. "So, to make her more comfortable, we put stage directions on the carpet."

Ophie was already fourteen years old at the time of my first visit. I learned that he had been a very pampered pooch, traveling everywhere with Tommy and sharing a tiny portion of whatever Tommy ate for years. That all changed a few months before when Ophie was diagnosed with heart disease. Although he took several medications to control his heart failure, his chronic cough continued to be a problem.

There were times when Ophie would cough all night, and neither he nor Tommy got any sleep. I'm not sure how that affected Tommy, but often Ophie wouldn't eat or drink the next day, and when you only weigh five pounds and take a diuretic, dehydration is a concern. I treated him with a small volume of subcutaneous electrolyte fluid and an appetite stimulant to put him back on track. But as Ophie worsened over time, his severe coughing episodes would cause his trachea, his windpipe, to collapse on itself, which would make it even harder for him to stop coughing. Eventually, he was taking narcotic cough suppressants that made him eat even less.

On one of my visits to treat him for his usual upset stomach, things seemed different. Ophie had a fever, and he cried when I palpated his abdomen. A blood test confirmed that he had pancreatitis, inflammation of his pancreas, a potentially serious condition. Although in theory, pancreatitis is treatable with fluids and supportive care, some patients don't respond and die from this disease.

"Tommy," I said, "Ophie is much sicker than usual. His pancreatitis must be treated aggressively with intravenous fluids, which needs to be done in the hospital. Ophie is tiny, and he has congestive heart failure, so there must be twenty-four-hour monitoring to balance his fluid needs and make sure his heart doesn't get overloaded."

"Absolutely not!" said Tommy.

A lot of clients say "No!" to a hospital stay. They want their pets to feel safe and secure in the home environment. That's why my house call practice is appealing. But I wasn't equipped to do this kind of round-the-clock hospital care at home. I did my best to convince him, but I wasn't able to.

"Amy, I know Ophie is nearing the end of his life. I know for sure that I don't want him to pass alone in a hospital away from me. Do what you need to do to make him better but do it in my home."

If Tommy wouldn't take Ophie to a hospital, then the hospital would have to come to him. I had never done this before, but within a few hours, I had created a mini-hospital inside his apartment. I brought in the fluid pump, a central venous pressure system, and round-the-clock nurses. Ophie stayed in his own bed, on intravenous fluids and anti-nausea injections, all while having his blood pressure, blood glucose, heart and respiratory rates, and hydration status monitored 24/7 and all within the sight of Tommy.

After five days, Ophie stabilized, and we could dismantle our makeshift hospital. I saw the tiny Yorkie regularly from that point to manage his various conditions and symptoms. But even pampered little sweeties like Ophie are not immortal, and I knew his time was drawing near. Tommy would be devastated when his beloved pet of eighteen years eventually passed away.

"You need to adopt another dog," I urged Tommy. "Now."

He looked at me as if I were nuts.

"I think it will be good for Ophie to have a companion, and he can pass along to the next generation everything the pup needs to know to be your pet." I strongly believed all of that to be true, and I also knew that the pain and stress of losing Ophie would be easier for Tommy if he had another dog to focus his love and attention on.

Tommy said, "I don't know, Amy."

I kept up my adopt-a-pet campaign with Tommy for a couple of months while Ophie hung in. And, finally, in September of that year, he got Little Shubert, a Yorkie puppy. As frail as Ophie was, he did seem to enjoy having a new friend around the house.

"It's incredible," Tommy told me, excitedly. "Ophie is really teaching Little Shubert everything he needs to know. I can see Ophie training him."

Ophie must have known when he finished the job. He passed peacefully in October, one month after Little Shubert's arrival. In that short amount of time, Ophie passed to his baby brother everything he needed to know to be a part of this family, and Tommy was able to turn his huge spotlight of love onto Little Shubert.

Three months later, Tommy invited me to the closing night performance of his one man show, *Tommy Tune: White Tie and Tails*, at the Little Shubert Theatre. Steve and I were awed by Tommy's singing, dancing, and tapping to classics from the American Songbook. He invited us to join him at the after-party backstage, and Steve took a photo of me and Tommy together. Even in my highest heels, I only stood as high as his waist. We sat together with a glass of champagne, and Tommy told Steve that he would love me forever, especially because of my advice to bring in a little brother for Ophie.

Matters of life and death can be philosophical as well. Even if everything I know about medicine makes me conclude that my patient should be helped to pass peacefully, I must be sure that my clients are all in agreement. There may be regrets that they waited too long, but euthanasia cannot be taken back once it is done.

If I am in someone's home and ready to perform a humane euthanasia and they are at that moment not completely certain, I will pack my things and let them know we can come back another day. Sometimes, they call back and ask me to return that same day. That second time, they are ready.

I went to a lovely, airy, sunny apartment on the Upper East Side to meet a new client and patient. A uniformed Eastern European–accented housekeeper answered the door and told me, "Madam will be with you shortly." She led us to the living room couch in the next room and gestured for us to sit down while waiting.

Carida and I were on a very tight schedule that day, and I didn't really have time to wait for Madam. I needed to see the cat so that I could get to my following appointments on time. But not wanting to make a scene with a new client, I sat in the living room, twiddling my thumbs, waiting. I began to look around, noticing the art on the walls. It was a lovely collection of School of Paris paintings. Then I noticed the Judaica antiques and the bookshelf packed with Jewish authors.

A dashing older man came into the room and in an accented voice he said, "Pardon me, Doctor. I'm so sorry my wife has kept you waiting. She'll be with you right away."

I recognized him immediately. He was Elie Wiesel, a Nobel Peace Prize winner, the Romanian-born author of dozens of books, including *Night*, about his imprisonment at Auschwitz during the Holocaust. Elie Wiesel is often thought of as the world's conscience of the postwar age. I meet a lot of famous people in their homes as a house call vet, but I'd never felt so honored to meet someone as I did at that moment with Elie Wiesel.

Marion Wiesel appeared next, an elegant, silver-haired woman with a broad smile. She held out her hand for a firm shake and sat next to me on the couch. She told me all about her elderly cat, Pizzi. Although Pizzi was healthy now, she got stressed when she went to the vet's office, and so Mrs. Wiesel wanted Pizzi to have house calls. She had me come that day because she wanted Pizzi to meet me, and she wanted to get to know me herself before there were any issues. Even though I was going to be hopelessly late for the rest of the day, I remained talking to Mrs. Wiesel well beyond my usual allocated time. I enjoyed that first conversation with her, as I have all the others I've had with her through the years. And it was crystal clear how much she loved cats, especially this one.

I saw Pizzi every few months and periodically checked her kidney function, which was starting to deteriorate. I often said hello to Mr. Wiesel, and we occasionally briefly chatted, but I always dealt with Madam, whom I simply called Mrs. Wiesel.

By the end of the year, Pizzi had developed kidney disease. It progressed to the point that she required daily injections of electrolyte solution. Like so many of my patients with long-term chronic kidney problems, Pizzi stabilized for a while but her kidneys slowly got worse despite the treatments. This is a result of normal aging, and there is no cure.

In the third year following her diagnosis, Pizzi was no longer feeling well. Her quality days were fewer, and she no longer wanted to eat on her own. Mrs. Wiesel and I discussed whether I should put Pizzi to sleep. She asked me to come back the next day and speak with her entire family.

That conversation took place in the master bedroom, with Pizzi lying on her side in the center of the bed. I spoke while watching her shallow breathing.

"From what you have told me and what I see now, I don't think

Pizzi has any quality of life," I said. To me, that is the key question, whether the pet is suffering, whether it has any quality of life.

The room was silent. And then, although he had not been part of our previous discussions, Mr. Wiesel now spoke, softly, looking at Pizzi. "Every single life," he said with emphasis on each word, "no matter what stage it is in, is precious." And then he looked up at Mrs. Wiesel, his son, and then at me. "Who are we to take a life?" asked this man whose adult life has been devoted to that very question.

And who was I to disagree with Elie Wiesel about the value of every single life?

But I did have an obligation, and so I continued. "Pizzi is going to die soon. I don't know how that's going to be. I don't know if she'll close her eyes and pass in her sleep or if it will be a struggle for her just to breathe. But what I do know is that I can help make the process of dying painless for her and for the people who love her."

I left the room for the family to discuss this agonizing question among themselves. After a few minutes, Mr. Wiesel called me back in and said, "We're ready to say goodbye."

I don't know what was said while I was out of the room, but if all life and all *of* life is precious, then I believe it is important that the end of life should be as easy and graceful as possible.

CHAPTER 17

Rescues, the Greatest Gift

Duchess, my first pet, was a rescue animal, just like every pet I've had after her.

Some clients of mine who have had purebred pets are hesitant to adopt a rescue animal. They say things like, "Something must be wrong with it because the previous owner gave it up."

This couldn't be further from the truth. Let me put some fears to rest about adopting a rescue. According to statistics from Best Friends Animal Society, a leading animal welfare organization working to end the killing of dogs and cats in America's shelters, animals are abandoned in two out of three cases because of *human* problems.* It's rarely about the animal's behavior. The most common causes of surrendering a pet to a shelter are, first, housing issues, then finances, the owner's death or illness, and only last, a poor pet-person connection.

---

* Best Friends Animal Society, "No-Kill 2025: The State of Animal Welfare Today," footnote 5, bestfriends.org/no-kill-2025/animal-welfare-statistics#5.

But even a bad fit doesn't mean a bad animal. For example, a rambunctious dog might not work for an elderly couple in the city but would be perfect for a family with young kids in the country. For these reasons, along with overbreeding and overpopulation, six million cats and dogs enter shelters every year, and sadly, nearly one million of them are euthanized, according to the American Society for the Prevention of Cruelty to Animals.*

I hope sharing the shocking statistics about unwanted animals that are ultimately euthanized because there's no home for them makes people realize how important it is to bring those numbers down. On the brighter side, four million animals *are* adopted from shelters each year,† including lots that I rehome to my own clients.

I've always believed that when you rescue a pet, *it knows* that it's been sought out and chosen and is forever grateful to you for it. The bond between a rescued pet and its person is incredibly strong. I can testify to it.

Michele Kleier had always gone to a high-end breeder for her Maltese dogs. After Daisy died, she was thinking about calling the same breeder to get another Maltese puppy.

At the same time, I knew that Rhoda, an elderly client of mine, couldn't continue caring for her beautiful Maltese, Tootsie. She'd been telling me this for a while but until now couldn't let her go. Now, she was ready.

"I think it's time," she told me.

"I know just the right family for Tootsie, and they will give her

---

* ASPCA, "Pet Statistics," www.aspca.org/helping-people-pets/shelter-intake-and-surrender/pet-statistics.

† ASPCA, "Pet Statistics," www.aspca.org/helping-people-pets/shelter-intake-and-surrender/pet-statistics.

the most wonderful life. I promise you, she will be a very happy dog, and she'll get the best of everything."

After hanging up with Rhoda, I called Michele. "I have your next dog. She's five years old and has been my patient since she was a puppy. She lives with an older woman who can't care for her any longer."

"Are you out of your mind?" she scoffed. "I'm not adopting someone else's dog," as if I was asking her to wear secondhand Bill Blass.

"No, Michele. This really is your dog." I just knew Tootsie and Michele were meant to be together. As a vet and pet matchmaker, I had the "yes" feeling. I'm not bragging, but my pet matchmaking instincts are very good.

I brought Tootsie to Michele's chaotic, loving home. She took one look at the dog, and said, "Okay, you're right. This is my dog."

Tootsie fit right in and immediately joined the Kleier pack, bringing its number up to three. And, just as I promised Rhoda, Tootsie had the best of everything for the rest of her life.

My client of over a decade, Nancy Shevell, was bereft after her beloved Jack Russell terrier died, and I encouraged her to get another pet. "We don't *replace* one dog or cat with another," I offered. "We just renew our love. And since love is infinite, you don't have to worry about it running out," I told her.

She listened to my advice, but she didn't take it. "I can't bring myself to get a new dog," she said. "When I'm ready, you'll hear from me."

For years, Nancy lived without a dog. She did manage to fall in love with another human, a lovely man named Paul, who was also a devoted dog person. He'd even written a song about his Old

English sheepdog, Martha, years ago when he was in a British rock band called the Beatles.

After the couple had been married for a few years, Nancy called me to say that she and her husband, Sir Paul McCartney, were ready to get a dog. "What breed should we get?" she asked.

"A rescue!" I replied instantly. "An animal that you bring home from a shelter knows it's been saved and will love you to bits. And what a wonderful message you two will be sending to the world that one of the most famous animal-loving people has chosen *to rescue* a dog. This is a message that needs to be heard, and you two are ideally suited to deliver it."

Sir Paul and Nancy took my advice and adopted Rose, a beautiful pit-bull Jack Russell terrier mix, and the three of them are devoted to each other to this day. As you can imagine, I look forward to every house call at this home. And the best news is that Nancy and Sir Paul were generous in publicizing Rosie's adoption, which I am sure increased pet adoptions around the world.

For whatever reason, adoptions are not for everybody. For example, I have clients who are devoted to particular breeds from specific breeders. No qualms there. Breeding purebred dogs is a centuries-old tradition, and quality breeders care about the essence of what a breed should be, what it should look like, what its function is, and what its best qualities are. And they keep their dogs healthy.

On the other hand, factory farming, also known as commercial breeding of animals or "puppy mills," comes with complete disregard for the health and temperament of these animals. This source of dog breeding is the bane of my existence.

Puppy mills, and that's who supplies pet stores, are not quality breeders. Their mission is simply to breed a dog as often and as cheaply as possible with little regard for proper health care and nutrition of either the mother or the offspring. They just try to get into the market as many animals as possible to cater to whatever the current breed fad is. Often, puppy-mill breeding focuses on one trait only, usually aesthetic, and disregards far more consequential traits, like temperament or increased risk of illnesses.

Factory-farmed dogs live in utterly appalling conditions. The dogs stay in small cages, often without proper food, basic vaccinations, grooming, or training. People see an adorable puppy in a pet shop window, buy it, but have no idea that it comes from a horrific past, often preloaded with costly high-maintenance physical issues and temperament problems that they are assuredly unprepared to deal with. Eventually, many change their minds and take their now-unwanted puppy-mill pet to a shelter because of these problems. Some of the dogs can be treated, rehabilitated, and adopted out, but sadly, some remain in small cages likely facing euthanasia.

Our animal-loving society needs to be aware that the puppy-mill industry fuels the huge numbers of animals in shelters, as well as ensuring the heartbreaking reality of their sad, short lives.

In many cases, I find that puppy-mill dogs are already sick when they are sent to pet stores. Then, in an effort to save money, pet stores often attempt to treat the animals themselves, usually causing the dog even more harm.

That's what happened to an adorable mini-dachshund puppy who wound up critically injured when he was given the wrong treatment by a penny-pinching pet store owner. The puppy was lethargic, and the store owner had seen a vet treat this condition many times, so he erroneously injected the puppy under its skin with an extremely concentrated dextrose sugar solution. But concentrated dextrose cannot be injected in this manner, and the result was massive destruction of the puppy's skin.

Within days, a large area of skin around the injection site turned black. The pet store owner wouldn't send the puppy to the local animal hospital when it needed only outpatient care, and now he certainly wasn't going to pay for the necessary hospitalization. Instead of veterinary care, he simply sent the little pup with one of his employees to the hospital to have it put down.

Carida was working her overnight shift at the Long Island hospital when the dachshund puppy was brought in. When she saw it, she asked if she could keep the puppy and the pet store employee said he didn't care as long as there was no bill to the store. She nursed the puppy during her shift that night and then brought him to City Pets the next morning.

She hadn't told me about the puppy, but the second I walked into my office, I knew something was wrong.

"Attas, I just didn't know what to do. I know it's a big ask, but you have to help him," she pleaded.

"Whoa, Carida, what's going on? Help who?"

"The most adorable dachshund puppy came into the hospital while I was on the overnight. They told us to put him to sleep. He's from the pet store, and they don't care what happens to these puppies. They just want to make money."

"Okay, so . . . help how?"

She hesitated, which was unusual for Carida, and then said, "He has no skin."

What?

She went back to her desk area and returned with a brown and white puppy. The puppy himself was brown, but all I could see of him was his long nose, legs, and tail, which was wagging up a storm. The rest of his body was swaddled in white bandages like a mummy. He was a three-pound, nine-week-old miniature dachshund. At this point, I didn't know the extent of his injuries, but I knew that at least his nose and tail worked.

I started to unwrap the bandages and Carida told me what she knew about his history.

Because he had a body bandage, I assumed he had a significant skin injury, but I was not prepared for what was unveiled. When I got to the last wrap of gauze, his devitalized skin was sticking to the bandage. It was much worse than I could have ever imagined.

"I'm not sure that there's anything I can do for this puppy," I said sadly to Carida.

Holding back tears, she said, "But look at his wagging tail. Look at his sweet face? Can't we just try?"

Heavy sigh. "Okay, okay," I said, watching his metronomic tail. "But if I feel he's suffering, I'm going to put him to sleep."

Since I had committed to him, our little puppy needed a name. We named him Dex because his injuries were a result of the dextrose injection he was improperly given.

His treatments included twice-daily antiseptic bathing, which he actually seemed to enjoy. After he was gently patted dry, I would rewrap him in sterile bandages so that once again only his head, legs, and tail were visible. *Those soulful eyes.* I started him on an oral antibiotic to prevent infection. Because he was so young and so small, I didn't have a lot of choices and I selected Clavamox, a penicillin-type drug that is both safe and effective for a very young puppy.

Each day, I repeated the whole process. Because his injuries were so dramatic, Steve suggested I photograph his progress daily. Initially, I wondered if treating him was the right thing to do, because Dex wasn't getting any better. But he was eating well, really liked the baths, and he didn't object to the occasional debridement (removal) of his necrotic skin. And his tail wouldn't quit. *How could he remain so happy?*

After two weeks of treatment, remarkably, pink granulation tissue was appearing, which meant healthy skin was growing back. And in a month, Dex was strong enough to have the remaining devitalized areas of skin surgically removed and the healthy skin edges sutured together. It was the surgical equivalent of connecting islands in an ocean with bridges. At the end of the second month, with two more surgical interventions, Dex had grown back healthy skin over his entire body and looked like a normal puppy. His recovery was amazing, like nothing I've ever seen.

Dex had many admirers, not only because of his remarkable recovery from this horrific injury but also due to his fabulous, always-happy attitude, which, given his circumstances, was even more remarkable. A nurse from the hospital was the lucky one who got to adopt him. Although we were all quite sad to say good-bye to our little Dex, he got a loving forever family. And we all got enormous satisfaction that we had saved this sweet, innocent dog's life.

Months after Dex went to his forever home, I attended a veterinary meeting sponsored by Pfizer, the drug company that manufactures Clavamox. At the meeting, Pfizer announced a case study competition where vets were invited to report on an interesting case in which Clavamox was used to treat and cure a patient. The grand prize was a one-week trip to Hawaii and the opportunity to present the report at a veterinary conference in Maui. The deadline for entry was one year from the meeting.

After the meeting, I sat down at my computer and my fingers flew as I typed up Dex's case in just half an hour. I attached all the progress photographs and sent the case report electronically to Pfizer, a full year before the deadline.

Not twenty-four hours later, the Clavamox rep called my office offering to donate all the antibiotics needed for Dex's care. The next day, the head of Pfizer's veterinary department called to ask if she herself could adopt Dex. Clearly both were so moved by reading the beginning of the report when they contacted me, they didn't even finish the document and learn that Dex was long ago both cured and adopted.

I told Steve about the call, and he smiled and said simply, "I think you should go bathing suit shopping."

"Why?"

"You're going to win the grand prize. We're going to Hawaii!"

I won the competition. Our trip to Hawaii was fabulous, but the real prize was saving that sweet, deserving little dog's life and setting him up in his forever home. I would do it all over again, no question, with or without a grand prize. It was all about his wagging tail and those eyes.

The older I get, the more I believe that even bad things happen for a reason.

I was contacted about a geriatric pug who had a multitude of medical problems and had been abandoned at a local shelter. The people at the shelter knew of my passion for pugs and my commitment to helping homeless animals, and they hoped that I'd take his case.

His medical problems were those of neglect. He had a skin infection, ear infections, a fungal infection in the folds of his face and between his toes. His breath was horrible from rotting teeth, and he walked with a terrible limp. He had not been neutered.

After a few weeks of antibiotics, a dentistry procedure to extract fifteen teeth, and a neuter, Pugly became a presentable dog. He was still geriatric, with a limp from arthritis and a broken right front leg that hadn't healed properly. The leg didn't hurt him, but he did walk funny. There was nothing else I could do for him medically.

Now, I needed to find Pugly a home. This was not going to be easy to do. Who wanted an old, limping, toothless dog?

Mr. Genovese, one of my elderly clients, lived alone in Greenwich Village with his fourteen-year-old dog, Holly. "Holly's not acting right," he said. "She has no appetite and is coughing a lot. I'm worried about her."

This combination of symptoms suggested a bad problem like heart or lung disease. Holly's X-ray showed a large amount of fluid in her chest. I drained the fluid from her lungs and took another X-ray. That scan plainly showed a large lung tumor. The lab results confirmed that it was cancer. I hated giving Mr. Genovese this news. At eighty, he had many medical problems himself, including severe arthritis that made it hard for him to walk without a cane or walker.

"I'm so very sorry, but there's nothing more we can do for Holly," I said.

"I guess that's it then. We have to say goodbye to her," he said.

I went to his rent-stabilized, one-bedroom apartment, and together we put his beloved companion to sleep. Mr. Genovese acted bravely, but I knew that losing Holly was traumatic for him. I hated to leave him that day, knowing that as soon as the door closed behind me, Mr. Genovese would be alone in this world. He had no family and many of his friends were either dead or had left the City.

I called him the next day to see how he was doing. "Hello, Dr.

Amy." He sounded much older than yesterday. "Hold on for a second, Doc." When he came back on the line, his speech was much better. I realized he'd put me on hold to insert his false teeth. "I'm doing okay, but it's very hard being here without Holly. I keep looking for her on the couch and then remembering she's gone."

"I want to talk to you about this dog I've been treating," I said. "He's an old pug who was abandoned and needs a home. It's not going to be easy, because he can't walk so well, and he's lost most of his teeth." But again, my pet matchmaking sense said "yes."

"Bring him over," he said bravely. "Let's have a look at him."

It took only a few minutes for Mr. Genovese to decide to keep Pugly, and the dog seemed very comfortable both in the apartment and with Mr. Genovese. I checked in with the pair the next day. "I think we're going to be fast friends," said Mr. Genovese. "We have a lot in common. We both can't walk, we both have no teeth, and we both snore. I guess it's meant to be that we live together."

I smiled.

As so often with cases like this, you have to wonder, who's really getting rescued?

CHAPTER 18

A Good Way to Heal

I can't tell you how many times someone has said to me after their pet has passed, "I will never have another pet again." I've said it myself. These words are said in the midst of such enormous grief that we feel the need to protect ourselves from ever feeling that pain again. I think that self-protection is part of our grieving process.

The appropriate amount of time before being open to loving a pet again differs for each person. Even my own broken heart has eventually been able to love again. And in my experience, the best way to heal is by rescuing a pet who needs you as much as you need them.

My beloved blind Bumper passed away peacefully at home with us when he was fifteen. He died in Steve's arms. Although we knew he had had a long and wonderful life, Steve and I had a great deal of difficulty coping with our grief. We had recently gotten married, and our newlywed bliss was cut short by our loss. Our new home was suddenly very empty.

I buried myself in work since I can't dwell in sadness when I am so fully engaged. But when I returned home from work each day, exhausted, I walked around the apartment absent-mindedly looking for little Bumper. I often thought that I saw him sleeping next to the wall, but it would turn out to be just a pair of shoes or even a shadow. After so many years of being together, his presence was programmed into my brain.

A year later, even though I still missed Bumper terribly, I realized that I was now missing having a dog in my life. When I started a conversation about getting one, Steve immediately changed the subject. After a few attempts, I realized that my new husband and I were not on the same page of a major life issue.

"Steve," I asked, "when do you think we might get another dog?"

"I can't. I honestly think I might never have another pet. I can't go through that pain again," Steve said tearing up. He added what he'd heard me say many times, "If everything goes right, your beloved pet is going to pass away before you do, and that is not anything I want to experience again."

More months went by, and my heart continued to feel very empty without a dog. I shared Steve's fear of future pain, but I also knew that the years of love and companionship were worth it. I pushed a little harder. When he didn't agree, I told him I *had to* have a dog.

"I understand," he said to me. "If you need to have a dog, then I think we should get one for you. But you must understand that I am not ready to love like that again. I simply can't let myself."

I appreciated his understanding of my need and his compromise.

"I won't do anything unless you're in agreement, but I'm going to put out some queries about rescue pugs," I said. He nodded his agreement.

Every pet I ever had has been a rescue, and I was going to do that again, although rescue pugs are not easy to come by. I knew that it might take months or even years to find the right dog and that would give Steve a chance to warm up to the idea.

To my surprise, a week after I put out some feelers, I got a call about Scruff, a rescue pug being fostered in an apartment close to where we lived.

When I got home from work that night, I made Steve a gin and tonic and said, "Great news, sweetie."

He looked at me and didn't say a word. He could see *pug* written all over my face.

"I'm going to meet the dog," I said. "I won't make any decisions without you."

"We are partners in everything, so if this is a possibility and you are going to meet this dog, I'll go with you." He gave me a look that said how much he loved me, and I kissed him.

"I am going to meet him tomorrow morning at seven before house calls," I said.

"I hate the timing, but okay," he consented.

I quickly refilled his gin and tonic and kept it topped off all night.

At seven a.m., we knocked on the door of the foster home and heard the piercing shrill of Scruff's barking. When the door opened, we could see that he was a tumbleweed with legs. A leaping, yipping ball of energy, he tore around madly, chasing his tail and barking incessantly. He didn't engage with us at all. We stayed with him for half an hour and then I had to excuse myself to get to work on time. Steve surprised me by asking the foster family if he could stay for a while longer. He wanted to get to know Scruff a little better and asked if he could take him for a walk. Some of Steve's favorite times with Bumper were their long walks around the neighborhood and in Central Park.

We didn't have a chance to speak all day, but when we were together that evening at home, he said, "Amy, I've been thinking."

That doesn't sound good.

"Scruff is a beautiful dog, but he is not our dog. I didn't feel a connection with him. I took him for a long walk and tried to get him to engage with me—just look up at me—and he wasn't interested. He needs a home in the country with kids and a big yard. I'm sorry."

Steve was right. In truth, I hadn't felt any bond with Scruff either. "I agree," I told him.

"But this experience made me realize that I do want a dog again," he continued. "I think I *need* one, just as much as you do. Just not Scruff. Is that okay?"

"Totally okay," I said. The wrong dog led Steve to make the right decision, and I was relieved. I owed Scruff for this and eventually paid him back by matching him with a big, rowdy family in upstate New York.

"One more thing," he said. "It might feel like the right time, but you can't force love. Love has to find us in its own time. Just like we did with each other."

A month later, I got a call from the manager of American Kennels on Lexington Avenue. The store had been there for years. When I was a child, my parents brought me there to watch the puppies tumbling around in the window. I'd had no idea then that pet store puppies were supplied by puppy mills that overbred dogs and didn't give them proper care. As a kid, I just saw cute puppies.

But as a grown-up veterinarian, I'd vowed to have nothing to do with such establishments.

I knew Mike, the manager of the store, and he wasn't a bad guy. He cared about the puppies and treated them well. As an employee of the store, he had to follow the owner's rules. But today he wanted to break one of those rules, and that was why he called me.

"Amy, I need your help. We have a four-month-old black pug in the store," he said. "We just figured out that he's totally blind. He is an amazing puppy but now that we know he's blind, he can't be sold, and he has to, well, go." Mike knew of my devotion to pugs, and he'd met blind Bumper. He was smart to have called me.

"Has to go" meant that the puppy was going to be euthanized.

"When?" I asked.

"Today at five."

Oh my goodness. "I'll be there as soon as I can." Without hesitating, I instructed my driver to reroute and head straight to the pet shop. An hour later, I was heading home with a handsome, blind black pug puppy on my lap. I called Steve.

"Sweetheart, I met a pug today."

Short silence. "Okay," he replied. "What's wrong with him?" he asked.

"He's blind."

"And where is he now?" he asked, like the good lawyer he was.

"With me."

"Right. And where are you?"

"In the car. Almost at the building."

Steve was waiting on the sidewalk when we pulled up. As he opened the car door, I nervously handed him the puppy. Steve held him up to look at him, and the puppy immediately started to lick his face. We went upstairs, and all the while the puppy didn't stop licking Steve's face.

As Steve tells it, he continued to lick his face for the next fourteen years. Steve was in love. We named him Leonardo for a multitude of reasons, but mainly because he had the heart of a lion and the sight of a master artist.

We never stopped missing Bumper, but something amazing happened when Leonardo came into our lives. When we thought about Bumper now, we were able to focus on our wonderful memories instead of our grief. Leonardo, our precious, rescued, also-blind puppy was already mending our broken hearts. We knew Bumper had sent him.

I've devoted my professional life to healing animals, with complete awe and appreciation for how our animals heal us. They make our hearts full, just by being near them. We feed and house them and easily give them our love, and *they give us everything they have in return*. What else do we owe our pets for their loyalty and companionship? Hardly anything at all in comparison: annual checkups and vaccines; medicine and supportive care when they're sick; and, when it's time, a humane passing. It's a great bargain. By doing these things, we fulfill our side of the unspoken agreement, to love and to care for them and to be loved and cared for *by* them, for as long as we get to be together. And in so doing, we make our homes—which are their entire worlds—the best place they could possibly be for both of us.

Acknowledgments

I've wanted to write this book for as long as I can remember. I have hundreds of stories from my decades of experiences—but how would I put them all together? And then I realized that, like everything else in my life that was difficult to do, I couldn't do it alone. I have so many people to thank who helped me pursue a career in veterinary medicine, start a unique practice, and ultimately write this book.

I must start with my family. My loving mom and dad could not have been more supportive of my dream to become a veterinarian and of my brother Lewis's dream to become a "people" doctor. Through the years, each of them played a part in getting me where I am, both figuratively and literally. Dad drove me to the Canadian border for a summer job on a dairy farm, and Mom and Lew drove me to my interview at Cornell University, where mom almost fainted during the tour when she caught site of a cow having surgery. When I first launched City Pets, they handed out leaflets at parties, helped with office work, and even took turns driving my team around Manhattan before I (thankfully) found a regular driver. I know how proud my dad would be if he were still with us and reading my book.

The first step in fulfilling my lifelong dream of becoming a veterinarian was meeting Dr. Jay Luger, the founder of the Forest Hills Cat Hospital, where I began volunteering as a teenager. Not only was he an excellent and compassionate veterinarian, but he was also a pioneer in starting the unique style of a feline-only practice. He also believed in a pushy fourteen-year-old kid who told him, "I have to be a vet."

City Pets wouldn't exist if it weren't for my team of coworkers, current and past. I must begin with George Simonoff, who instantly and selflessly helped me on that tumultuous, uncertain day one ("Tell me what I can do to help."). He has been one of my greatest supporters and closest friends ever since. Likewise, special thanks are due to my old and good friend Gene Solomon, my senior veterinarian when I first practiced on Park Avenue and my savior when I suddenly found myself hospital-less. Gene unhesitatingly came to my rescue at that moment, offering material and emotional support that continues to this day.

Thank you of course to my current team at City Pets, many of whom have been by my side for years and even decades. There is Dr. Danielle Dalton, my associate for more than twenty years, who treats every patient as if they were her own pet. My talented, compassionate technicians, Carida Fernandez and Jeanine Lunz, also with me for decades, who give one hundred percent to our furry patients and their families. Back at the office, a complex logistical command center, Elena Jones and James Warbritton not only compassionately handle the needs of our clients and their pets but also skillfully juggle their schedules. Thanks are due to Carlos

Lezama for getting us everywhere safely. Thank you also to Shari King, Ruvim Krupnikas, and Sandra Mack-Valencia, who were an essential part of the original team early on. And a very personal and special thank-you to Martha Ochoa, who started out as our assistant and became a member of our family.

A note of thanks to John Patch, who decades ago gave me an opportunity to tell some of my tales on his radio show, *Talking Pets*. It was the exercise of preparing a series of these weekly five-minute readings that helped me create the cache of early tales that would one day become the core of this book—and realize they were worth telling.

What veterinarian writes a book without thanking the great James Herriot? In my case, it's personal. I read *All Creatures Great and Small* when I was fourteen and was thrilled to meet him in Yorkshire when I was a veterinary student. Herriot's tales (his real name was Alf Wight) and love of both his patients and their people inspired me to set out on my own journey. With the inspiration of Herriot's books—a copy of *All Creatures* sits upright on my desk at all times—I began to write about those unique people, pets, and experiences. Visiting Thirsk, England, in 1999, for the opening of the Herriot Museum in the very building where he lived and practiced, I befriended both his daughter, Rosie, a retired physician, and his son, Jim, who worked with his father as a veterinarian. Having a personal tie through them to Herriot himself has helped keep his flame burning brightly inside of me.

I must also thank Valerie Frankel, who over many lunches, long phone calls, and a weekend of feeding baby chicks helped me turn my stories into *Pets and the City*. Her professional guidance has been essential, and I cherish her as a dear friend as well.

Thank you to my editor, Michelle Howry. I knew from my first

Acknowledgments

Zoom call how much I would enjoy working with her, and I was right. She and the team at PRH, including Ashley Di Dio, Ashley Hewlett, Kristen Bianco, and Shina Patel, have been so supportive.

A special thank-you to David Black, my friend, fellow dog lover, and agent. He signed on to this project when I really needed him with a promise to always be there for me. I am forever grateful.

My own very special pets—all pugs except for my barn cat, Mieskeit, who got me through a tough summer and many years thereafter—must be thanked. Not only have they enriched my life, they taught me real compassion. Through the years when each of them were seriously ill, I was forced to turn from veterinarian into pet mom—I learned to be a better vet from being on the other side.

From Duchess (my first pug who showed me how deeply I love dogs) to Bumper (the blind pug I rescued from the tree in front of the University of Pennsylvania Vet School), to the regal Leonardo (who truly had "The Force" and could hike an icy mountain path without a leash), to Winston (a pug puppy so sick and tiny that Carida brought him to me nestled in a backpack, and when he was cured I loved him so much I had to keep him)—each dog was so precious to me. In the years that followed, as those dogs passed away, we were joined by Cleopatra (an elegant, emotive adult black pug who my husband called his girlfriend), and Hermite (whose name was inspired by a hermit crab, because when she first came to us she was so frightened she would hide under her bed and walk around with it on her back). Hermite's name eventually evolved into "Meatball," just because.

During the writing of this book, our Cleopatra passed away at age sixteen, and tragically, three months later to the day, little Meatball passed away from a severe illness just two weeks after her ninth birthday. We know she just couldn't live without her big sister. And Steve and I are now having the same trouble, deeply aware of both missing souls every minute of the day. As I write this, for the first time in my life I do not have a pet, and as a result, also for the first time, my life is not complete. I know that there will be a rescue someday, but my broken heart must start to heal first.

I have left mentioning my husband, Steve, for last because I have so many things to thank him for. For more than thirty years he has been my partner and my best friend. We share our love of travel, food, wine, theater, music, books, and, of course, animals. Animals of all kinds. Domestic and wild. Here and gone. Steve is my biggest supporter, and he encourages me to pursue anything I want to do, telling me that of course I can do it. And I can—particularly knowing that he will always be by my side. And when I come home from work and tell him, "You won't believe what happened today!," he makes me sit and write down the stories. He reads (and edits) everything I write and makes it so much better. I am so lucky to have found and be with the love of my life.

And, of course, it was a dog who brought us together.